Beyond the
Water Towers

The unfinished revolution in mental health services 1985-2005

Edited by   Andy Bell

Peter Lindley

©The Sainsbury Centre for Mental Health 2005

ISBN: 1 870480 64 3

Published by

The Sainsbury Centre for Mental Health
134-138 Borough High Street
London SE1 1LB

Tel: 020 7827 8300
Fax: 020 7403 9482
www.scmh.org.uk

The Sainsbury Centre for Mental Health (SCMH) is a charity that works to improve the quality of life for people with severe mental health problems. It carries out research, development and training work to influence policy and practice in health and social care. SCMH was founded in 1985 by the Gatsby Charitable Foundation, one of the Sainsbury Family Charitable Trusts, from which it receives core funding. SCMH is affiliated to the Institute of Psychiatry at King's College, London.

A charitable company limited by guarantee registered in England and Wales no. 4373019

Charity registration no. 1091156

Design by Intertype
Printed by Stephens & George, UK

Cover photography by Alice Troun...

Contents

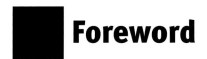

Foreword

Matt Muijen

This book provides a detailed overview of the developments in mental health care during the 20 years the Sainsbury Centre for Mental Health (SCMH) has been in existence, and illustrates well the tremendous transformation that has taken place over that time. It also demonstrates, by the breadth of subjects covered and the variety of backgrounds and perspectives of its contributors, how wide ranging, inclusive and ambitious the mental health field has become. It would have been quite unthinkable 20 years ago to publish a book on mental health care covering mental well being alongside hospital care, and putting the contributions of service users on an equal footing with those of psychiatrists.

It is difficult to overstate the scale of changes in mental health care across the UK, whether benchmarked against local or international standards. In the mid-1980s, mental health services in the UK relied on paternalistic care that was mostly hospital-based, lagging well behind reforms in several other countries around the world. I remember how embarrassing it was to lecture about the state of mental health services at international conferences in those days. Not any longer. In a time span much shorter than it took to build the asylums in the 19th century, their closure programme has been almost completed. In contrast to many other countries, considerable investment has been made to provide alternatives, in the shape of a comprehensive range of community-based services. It may not be perfect, but at least much is there.

It is worth noting the extent to which changes were driven by centralised, top-down managerial processes rather than local clinical initiatives feeding upwards. This did not exclude the involvement of representatives in the formulation of the National Service Framework. My memory of this period, much of it as chief executive of The Sainsbury Centre for Mental Health, is one of constant meetings and surprisingly genuine opportunities for a broad range of stakeholders to influence the content of policies. Just getting service users, interest groups and psychiatrists around the table was an achievement at the time.

The development of community care brought out into the open the needs and wishes of service users and carers. Clinicians had to deal with problems beyond diagnosing and prescribing. A frustration both users and clinicians mentioned was the impermeable boundaries between public service sectors such as social services, education, social security and various health care silos. The gradual steps to integrate these essential service components by introducing national legislation and freedoms for local initiatives changed the scope of mental health care. I remember a Secretary of State for Health less than 10 years ago stating that any structural integration between the centrally accountable NHS and locally accountable social services was unthinkable. We have indeed moved a long way in a short time.

A consequence of community care, addressed in several chapters, is the inevitable focus of mental health care on social and political issues. In the past, when patients were cared for in large institutions, culture, ethnicity and class could be ignored. Now, working with people in their own environments, mental health practitioners are faced with the consequences of stigma, discrimination and inequality. Lack of employment opportunities, over representation of minorities in prisons and special hospitals, unfair variations in accessibility and quality of care, and racism are some of the consequences which are mentioned frequently in this book. Training has prepared staff poorly to deal with such issues. It is surprising in retrospect how little thought was given to the changing roles and competencies of staff when they moved from an institutional setting to independent working in community settings. SCMH was a pioneer in this area, as described in this book, and it is promising that some of its future priorities are focusing on these challenges.

The history of mental health care tends to focus on services for people with severe and enduring conditions. The prevalence of anxiety and depression has probably always been high, but has not been seen as a responsibility of specialist mental health services until relatively recently. Now people demand interventions, often of a sophisticated nature, but the competence and capacity of services is insufficient. Whereas in the past this group was dismissed as 'the worried well', it is now recognised that these conditions carry a massive human and economic burden. The prevention and treatment of such conditions is fast becoming the leading public health challenge in the developed world. Shifting the responsibility to unprepared general practitioners is not the answer. An interesting question is whether the voluntary sector and the user movement accept such public health challenges to be within their remit, or whether they will remain focused on the human rights agenda for the group of people suffering the greatest stigma and discrimination.

So what about the future? My prediction is that mental health care will take on a much broader remit, incorporating well being, prevention, treatment and recovery. The challenge will be to create a dynamic balance between improving the mental well being of the population, preventing mental health problems in groups at risk and treating and integrating people with mental health problems into society. An associated challenge is how to create a meaningful continuum between these very different approaches, without dumping it into the lap of agencies who are either under resourced or incompetent. Key to any success will be how we tackle stigma and discrimination, issues that have affected all aspects of mental health.

Throughout its history, SCMH has played a very active part in all these areas. It has contributed to policy, and produced influential research reports on subjects such as assertive outreach, hospital care, workforce, services for Black people and mental health promotion. During its history, the quality of care provided by mental health services has been transformed. Whether there is an association between the two is an interesting question that I feel poorly qualified to answer, although I have an opinion. But SCMH can pride itself on having positioned itself consistently in the right places. It is also well placed for the future, possessing the right competences for the challenges I have identified. It continues to receive committed support from people with vision and a strong belief about the injustice of the fate of people with mental health problems in this world. Despite all the improvements over the last 20 years, such challenges remain.

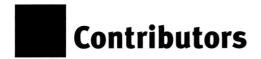
Contributors

Andy Bell is Director of Communications at the Sainsbury Centre for Mental Health. He was previously head of public affairs at the King's Fund, an independent health charity.

Dr Jed Boardman is Consultant Psychiatrist and Senior Lecturer in Social Psychiatry at South London and Maudsley NHS Trust and the Institute of Psychiatry, King's College London. He is also Senior Policy Advisor to the Sainsbury Centre for Mental Health.

Peter Campbell is a mental health system survivor. He has received services for over 35 years and was a founder member of Survivors Speak Out (1986) and Survivors' Poetry (1991). He worked for many years with pre-school children. Since 1990 he has been working as a freelance trainer and writer in the mental health field. He was born and raised in Scotland, lives in Cricklewood, north west London and supports Hendon FC.

Dr Alan Cohen was a GP for 25 years in Mitcham, prior to joining Kensington and Chelsea PCT in April 2004, as Clinical Director. He also works as Director of Primary Care at the Sainsbury Centre for Mental Health and chairs the London Development Centre for Mental Health, one of the eight regional development centres of the National Institute for Mental Health in England (NIMHE). He continues in active general practice in North Kensington.

Elizabeth Gale is the Director of **mentality**, the first national team dedicated solely to the promotion of mental health, at the Sainsbury Centre for Mental Health. She is one of the founding members of **mentality**, established in 2000. Previously she managed the policy programme for the Health Education Authority's (HEA) Mental Health Team working on national and international programmes. Before the HEA she worked at the Mental Health Foundation where she concentrated on the rights of people with learning disabilities and those who misuse substances. Her academic background is in law and sociology and she has a keen interest in the human rights and civil liberties agenda.

Prof Howard Goldman is Professor of Psychiatry at the University of Maryland School of Medicine. He also advises the trustees of the Gatsby Charitable Foundation on mental health issues.

Angela Greatley is Chief Executive of the Sainsbury Centre for Mental Health, where she was Director of Policy between 2002 and 2004. Previously she was Fellow in Mental Health at the King's Fund, from 1997, where she managed a major Mental Health Inquiry investigating the extent to which needs and services in London have changed over the last five years, and co-ordinated a programme designed to pilot three new assertive outreach teams for people with serious mental health problems in the capital. She began her NHS career working in community health councils and has been an elected member of a London local authority. She worked in a variety of NHS service management posts and led the community care programme at the North East Thames Regional Health Authority before becoming Director of Commissioning and Deputy Chief Executive in a London health authority.

Dr Bob Grove joined the Sainsbury Centre for Mental Health in 2003 to lead the Employment Programme. He began working in the mental health and employment field in 1985, and was the founding Director of Richmond Fellowship Employment and Training (RFET). After leaving RFET in 1998 he worked at the Centre for Mental Health Services Development at King's College London leading a programme of consultancy, research, policy and service development. He continues with these activities at SCMH and is currently seconded part-time to the Department of Health, working with the Department for Work and Pensions on the Incapacity Benefit Reform Pilots.

Dr Frank Keating is a Senior Research Fellow at the Sainsbury Centre for Mental Health, where he works as a member of the 'Breaking Circles of Fear' implementation team. This project aims to improve and develop mental health services for African and Caribbean communities. Frank takes a lead on evaluation and research in this project. Frank was lead author of the report *Breaking Circles of Fear: A review of the relationship between mental health services and African and Caribbean communities.*

Peter Lindley is Deputy Director of Practice Development and Training at the Sainsbury Centre for Mental Health. His recent work has included the *Capable Practitioner Framework* and the development of the *Ten Essential Shared Capabilities for Mental Health Practice*. He is particularly interested in approaches to teaching and learning that emphasise the lived experience of service users and carers, and that bridge the training and practice divide. He is also a Visiting Professor at Middlesex University.

Dr Matt Muijen is Regional Advisor for Mental Health at the World Health Organisation in Europe. Before that, he was Chief Executive of the Sainsbury Centre for Mental Health between 1989 and 2004. Matt worked as a practising Clinical Psychiatrist and researcher prior to joining SCMH.

Dr Steve Onyett is Senior Development Consultant for the National Institute for Mental Health in England development centre for the south west (NIMHE-SW) and Visiting Professor at the Faculty of Health and Social Care at the University of the West of England. He moved to the south west in 1998 from South Kent where he was Head of Clinical Psychology. His previous roles included being the founding team manager of an inner-London community mental health team providing assertive community treatment. Most recently he has been working with Carol Borrill on the development of the training pack to support the Leadership Centre's 'Effective Teamworking and Leadership in Mental Health' programme.

Michael Parsonage is an economist working at the Sainsbury Centre for Mental Health on a consultancy basis. He previously worked at the Department of Health and HM Treasury.

Malcolm Philip is Director of Workforce Development at the Sainsbury Centre for Mental Health. He has 18 years experience of Human Resources, 16 with the NHS, in acute care and in mental health. After a broad range of roles within Human Resources and having completed his MA in 1994, he became Director of Personnel for the Bethlem and Maudsley NHS Trust for nearly five years. As the Director of Personnel he focused on organisational development and strategic Human Resources. In 1999, he moved into research and consultancy work. He ran his own independent consultancy focusing on strategic Human Resources and organisational development. He was Human Resources Consultant with the Sainsbury Centre for Mental Health, prior to becoming leader of their Workforce Development Unit, and does research for the Department of Health into the mental health workforce.

Prof David Pilgrim is Clinical Dean at the Teaching Primary Care Trust for East Lancashire, Visiting Professor at the Department of Primary Care, University of Liverpool, and Honorary Professor at the Postgraduate Medical School at the University of Central Lancashire. He trained as a clinical psychologist, completed a PhD on NHS psychotherapy, a Masters in Sociology and since has divided his time between NHS and academic activity.

Lesley Warner is a senior researcher at the Sainsbury Centre for Mental Health. Following mental health and general nurse training in the early 1970s, she worked as a community psychiatric nurse, CPN Team Leader and community mental health service manager. After posts as a research nurse and as a health visitor, she established a walk-in service for people with serious mental health and social problems before working on a project to improve access to health services for homeless people. Since joining SCMH in 1994 she has evaluated many services within the statutory and voluntary sectors including inpatient and community-based services, day care, support services, work projects and supported housing schemes. She has contributed to SCMH's nationally-focused work, including the National Visits undertaken jointly with the Mental Health Act Commission. She has been leading the research input to the 'Search for Acute Solutions' project, and is currently working on a study of how the Care Programme Approach is implemented for detained patients.

Dr Jennie Williams is a clinical psychologist with a long-standing commitment to getting inequality taken seriously by mental health services. She is Director of Inequality Agenda, which provides training and support to services throughout the UK for women who have mental health needs. She retains some responsibilities at the Tizard Centre, University of Kent, where she worked as a Senior Lecturer in Mental Health for over ten years. She contributes through Department of Health committees to the implementation of the National Women's Mental Health Strategy and to getting equality issues on the agenda of workforce planning.

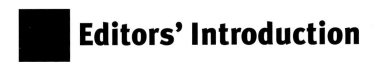

Editors' Introduction

Andy Bell and Peter Lindley

In 1985 most people who needed mental health care received it from services based in remote Victorian 'water tower' hospitals, or asylums. Thankfully this is no longer the case and, just two decades on, a much wider range of options is now available. Many people will receive the help that they need in or close to their own homes while the 'water tower' hospitals of old have been sold off or demolished.

There is no doubt that mental health services have changed for the better since 1985. There is also little doubt that services will continue to develop and change as service users and carers continue to articulate their views of what they need, and as knowledge of 'what works' continues to emerge. Yet there are also major concerns. For example, acute hospital care may have changed beyond recognition since 1985, but it is still in a state few would find acceptable. And there are threats on the horizon that could reverse much of the progress that has been made in the past two decades – foremost among them proposals to reform mental health law.

This book is published to mark the 20th anniversary of the Sainsbury Centre for Mental Health (SCMH). It looks at some of the most significant developments in mental health services since SCMH became active in 1985, at the time as the National Unit for Psychiatric Research and Development – the name changed to the Sainsbury Centre for Mental Health some years later.

The authors were selected on the basis of their track record of achievements in their field. Many either work at or have worked with SCMH during the past two decades. We asked each of them to review the most important changes in mental health services in their topic area over the past 20 years, to consider the current situation and to identify the key challenges for the future. The result is a comprehensive account of the state of the nation's mental health services that lays out a clear agenda for future development priorities.

Two chapters, by David Pilgrim and Peter Campbell, provide a powerful overview of the growth in the voice of mental health service users since 1985 – arguably the most exciting, relevant and challenging development in the entire field of mental health. Their chapters provide testimony to the emergence of a powerful service user movement that has had an enormous impact on the shape and delivery of mental health services, yet which still faces enormous challenges in a service where power is still unequally distributed. From a handful of isolated groups in the mid 1980s the movement has grown to encompass well over 500 local groups throughout the UK. It is difficult to imagine a development in service provision, an innovation in education and training or a new direction of any kind in mental health services that would not include service user participation.

Jed Boardman gives an overview of mental health policy over the past 20 years and notes some of the key changes that have taken place to support the move from institutional-based services to the development of community care. The major shift in national policy since 1985 has been the erosion of a post-war consensus and optimism, leading to policies that pay increasing attention to control and public safety.

Lesley Warner chronicles the development of acute care from 1985, when most people looking for help with acute distress could expect to be treated as an inpatient in a Victorian 'water tower' hospital, to the present day when a much wider range of options would be available or under development in their locality. Such services could include crisis resolution teams, crisis houses, partial hospitalisation, early intervention services, assertive outreach teams and multidisciplinary community mental health teams, provided by a combination of health, social care and voluntary sector organisations.

Two chapters focus on the vital issue of the key resources that make mental health services work: staff and money. Malcolm Philip focuses on the development of a workforce capable of providing modern mental health services. He describes the emergence of the current workforce crisis and the many challenges involved in creating a workforce for the future that will enable services to deliver the support that users and carers need.

In examining the mental health economy, Michael Parsonage argues that while expenditure on mental health services has increased considerably in the last two decades, the infrastructure to support services remains a major weakness. Constant reorganisations and a lack of investment in information technology, for example, have undermined the ability of services to meet people's needs. Future investment in mental health care, he argues, should be focused on these areas, as well as on improving direct service delivery.

Alan Cohen traces the development of primary care's role in mental health services. He shows how changes in mainstream health policy, such as the creation of fundholding, and subsequently of primary care trusts, has affected the way GPs and their colleagues offer support to people with mental health problems. He argues that it is only since 1999 that there have been any policies for primary mental health care, as a result of which real progress is now being made in practice.

One of the most important developments of the past 20 years has been the creation and proliferation of community care services. Steve Onyett examines how the role of the mental health team has been fundamental to the development of community services and shows that much still needs to be done to help them to function as teams and to work around the needs of service users.

Elizabeth Gale and Bob Grove emphasise the critical importance of a thorough understanding of the social, economic and political environments for every aspect of mental health practice. In addition, they describe how the importance of the social context for mental health has expanded over the last two decades in three main ways: recognition of the impact of social exclusion and isolation on mental health and well being; a growing understanding of the importance of tackling stigma and discrimination; and the embedding of mental health promotion and the enhancement of public mental health in tackling wider health inequalities. Yet, as the chapter shows, putting these understandings into action remains at an early stage of development.

Frank Keating and Jennie Williams examine one of the most neglected issues in mental health practice: inequalities. They argue that while gender, class and 'race' are now widely understood as important sources of social inequality, mental health services are poorly placed to address them and may actually help to perpetuate them. They set out a new agenda – critical for the next 20 years – to address this problem.

Howard Goldman, Professor of Psychiatry from the University of Maryland in the USA, is uniquely well placed to provide a perspective from America through his continued involvement with SCMH from the very early days and through his many visits to the UK. His chapter presents some observations from "across the pond" and reviews the similarities and differences between mental health services in the US and the UK, with a special focus on the role of mental health authorities and the evolving nature of stewardship for mental health services.

Finally, Angela Greatley examines what all these developments mean for the future. She argues that, while the past 20 years has seen a revolution in the way people with mental health problems are supported by public services, there is still much to be done. The key challenges, among many, will be to address inequalities in mental health care, to change the way mental health services work to support people in all aspects of their lives and to promote recovery in its fullest sense.

1 Protest and Co-option
– The voice of mental health service users

David Pilgrim

Introduction

In the last 20 years, the voice of the mental health service user has become more evident in academic studies of mental health, policy statements and in local service documentation. This chapter explores a tension between the service user perspective as an expression of protest and as a management resource. This tension is both evident and predictable. The notion that the personal accounts of people with mental health problems should be valued *collectively* has two different sources, each with distinct interests and ideologies. On the one hand 'experts by experience' have been part of a new social movement of disaffected service users attacking psychiatric theory and practice. On the other hand, the oxymoron of a 'lay expert' has found its time and modern health and welfare bureaucracies now emphasise consumerism as a source of quality improvement.

What both of these sources have in common is that they place a value on the reported experience of those who have been in contact with specialist mental health services. The mental health service user movement and user involvement in service improvement initiatives have overwhelmingly represented people who might variously be described as having 'serious and enduring mental health problems', 'severe mental illness' or simply as being 'mad'. However, the great bulk of people who are acknowledged to have mental health problems are treated in primary care. The voices of these, who have never entered an inpatient facility or even seen a specialist mental health worker, are barely represented in the discourse of *either* the users' movement or of users' views of services.

Mental health service users can be framed as patients, survivors, consumers or providers (Rogers & Pilgrim, 2001). In this chapter, only two of these are explored: survivors and consumers. Also, there is no space here to disentangle the confusing but common managerial amalgam of the 'views-of-users-and-carers'. When consulted, users and their significant others share some common concerns but they also disagree with one another on priorities and some fundamentals.

The voice of protest

The growth in the mental health service users' movement since the 1970s has been recorded by a number of commentators (Haafkens et al.,1986; Burstow & Weitz, 1988; Chamberlin, 1977; Rogers & Pilgrim, 1991; Crossley & Crossley, 2001). During the 1970s, the Dutch and American survivors' movements gained national and State recognition. By 1977, 35 organisations were recognised in the Netherlands. Organised patient pressure in the USA resulted in funding for research and for mental health services to be run exclusively by patients (Campbell & Schraiber, 1989). From the 1980s onwards similar developments took place in the UK.

User dissatisfaction reached such a point that, in terms of numbers and organisations, it constituted a mature 'new social movement'. A social movement can be defined as a loose network of people that actively resists established dominant forms of power or pursues cultural or social change (Toch, 1965). Social movements are characterised by mass mobilisation (e.g. demonstrations) and for the most part act outside of formal organisations and bureaucratised pressure groups and charities.

'New' social movements can be distinguished conceptually from the traditional labour movement in that they are not linked to protest and analysis of oppression in the work-place. New social movements seek to establish new agendas and conquer new territory (Habermas, 1981). Many, but not all, are built upon a shared oppressed identity (e.g. the Women's Movement and Gay Liberation). For this reason, new social movements have been associated with 'identity politics'. However, some are not built on a common identity but on a common just cause (e.g. Animal Rights and the Ecology Movement).

The mental health service survivors' movement fits broadly within this new pattern of political radicalism. It is characterised by opposition to expert medical knowledge and a form of politics based on an identity derived from mental health problems and contact with specialist services. Survivors' groups have shared several concerns highlighted previously by critical professionals during the 1960s ('anti-psychiatry'). Whereas that critique was highly intellectual and came from professionals themselves, the more recent one has come from service users directly and is less theoretically oriented and more concerned with direct action.

The mental health service users' movement has emerged from the previously atomised voices of lone mental patients. The transformation has led to a collective voice of shared resistance and demands for change. Changes in the status of the personal voice of the mental patient became evident after the Second World War. In the face of a discreditable identity of the mental patient, which prevailed in the 1950s and 1960s, the Mental Patients Union and other user groups in the 1970s strived to be assigned an authentic say.

A shift to a more collectivised voice is clearly evident since the 1980s. Users' experiences are wedded now to broader social groupings and issues (e.g. gender and sexual abuse).

The agenda of activism contributes explicitly to the discourse of political activism and resistance on the one hand and the development of alternative ways of managing 'madness' on the other. The 'lived experience' and voice of users are combined to produce an emancipatory way of dealing with mental suffering. This combination is evident, for example, in the way in which the Hearing Voices Network embraces and makes the connections between the social and the therapeutic:

> *"People who hear voices and their families and friends can gain greater benefits from de-stigmatising the experience, leading to a greater tolerance and understanding. This can be achieved through promoting more positive explanations, which give people a more positive framework for developing their own ways of coping and raising awareness about their experience in society as a whole."* (http://www.hearing-voices.org/)

The survivors' literature emphasises the oppression suffered by psychiatric patients, though the source of this is ambiguous. The person has 'survived' their mental health problems, their experience of psychiatric services and their general social exclusion.

Sometimes the survivors' movement is also described as an 'opposition movement' (Haafkens *et al.*, 1986). Although they make demands about citizenship, much of the anger and debates of disaffected patients focus on disappointments or frustrations about the psychiatric profession and mental health services. This is exemplified in the title, *Shrink Resistant: the Struggle Against Psychiatry in Canada* (Burstow & Weitz, 1988).

Given this disaffection about psychiatry and mental health services, the term 'user' is problematic, because patients do not necessarily view services as being 'of use', especially given the common scenario of involuntary contact. How can the notion of 'service' be justified when it is imposed – a 'service' to whom? In what sense do people who have contact with the mental health system against their will 'use' that system? Can a person validly use something that is forced upon them?

A number of themes can be identified from the narratives offered by patients and ex-patients:

❖ **The opposition to coercion**
   The focus here is on the way in which people with mental health problems are segregated forcibly from society.

❖ **The opposition to compulsory treatment**
   As well as the issue of compulsory detention, compulsory treatment is also opposed. Indeed the notion of medical treatment is inherently problematic if it is imposed. Assaults on resistant bodies are cast as 'treatment' because the State delegates lawful powers to professionals. Similarly what is solitary confinement in prison becomes 'seclusion' in mental health services. The users' movement seeks to expose the mystification of these oppressive practices carried out under the cloak of medical paternalism.

❖ **The opposition to psychiatric diagnosis**
This varies in its salience but many patients resent the application of a medical diagnosis to a problem they prefer to frame in biographical, social or spiritual terms.

❖ **The demand for greater treatment choice**
This relates to the dominant use of physical treatments in psychiatry. Users demand a greater choice of treatment responses than are on offer. Common demands are for psychosurgery and electroconvulsive therapy (ECT) to be outlawed and for psychological therapies to be more available.

❖ **The demand for greater citizenship**
This feature is shared with the physical disability movement. It is the one area of demand that lies outside complaints about psychiatry and specialist services, though the latter may still be criticised for not promoting social inclusion.

The co-opted voice: a resource for service quality assurance

As was noted in the introduction to this chapter, both the users' movement and the concern of those developing mental health services emphasised the view of one group of patients: those in episodic contact with specialist services. This has meant that the messages from the users' movement and the list recurring from consultation exercises with service users are remarkably similar. Much of the focus is on disappointment with specialist services, especially inpatient regimes.

Mental health services have always been, and have remained, associated with coercion and are dominated by forms of physical treatment. Indeed, over time this tendency has increased, for example, in the rising number of sections under the Mental Health Act. What patients generally want is non-coercive, holistic care. The latter term can sometimes be described as a 'psychosocial' or a 'bio-psychosocial' approach to care. At present, psychiatry and its adjacent group of mental health professions are found lacking in this regard.

According to users they do not regularly receive holistic, patient-centred care in inpatient settings. What they actually get are over-crowded holding centres with no time or space for individualised care plans or therapeutic interventions, except in the form of medication reviews. Inpatient services are noted for their 'non-therapeutic' character (SCMH, 1998) and for their habitual capacity to make patients feel worse rather than better in the wake of their admission (Mind, 2004).

The structure of mental health care in the last 20 years has amplified this tendency. With the closure of large mental hospitals, acute inpatient facilities have virtually abandoned their aspiration to be treatment facilities. They are now largely the recipients of coercively controlled patients, many of whom have concurrent problems ('co-morbidity', 'dual diagnosis'). The proportion of patients now detained involuntarily in these units is very high, as is bed occupancy. Twenty years ago, formal patients were in a minority. It remains a moot point though whether, even in those days of greater bed capacity, before the large hospitals closed, 'informal' patients, were truly voluntary (Rogers, 1993).

Proposals in the recent Draft Mental Health Bill to cast inpatient facilities in the role of assessment centres for the coercively detained may simply be formalising what they have now inevitably become.

In the early 1990s, Mind commissioned a large survey of patients' views of services (Rogers *et al.*, 1993). That snapshot occurred in the context of the large Victorian hospitals closing. The accounts given to us reflected the experiences of a unique cohort of patients who had been in both the old asylums and the District General Hospital acute units, which had emerged during the 1970s. The methodology was relatively unusual. A thousand patients collaborated with the survey but the extensive questionnaire was not completed individually. Instead it was done with the help of volunteers who elicited responses in a dialogue.

The survey found that:

❖ Mental health care was dominated by biological interventions. Nearly half of the sample had received ECT during their service contact, despite it ostensibly being a treatment of last resort.

❖ Only 60% received some form of psychological intervention during service contact, whereas 98% received drugs. Moreover, 85% had been taking psychiatric drugs for more than one year and nearly 40% of them for more than ten years.

❖ Over 60% of patients described the adverse effects of medication to be either 'severe' or 'very severe'.

❖ Only 10% of the patients interviewed actually saw their mental health problems in terms of mental illness. The rest gave a range of accounts for their difficulties. This highlights the tension between psychiatric codifications of mental abnormality and those provided by patients themselves.

❖ Patients preferred to be supported in non-hospital settings.

❖ Patients valued day care but not because of the service claims made by managers about treatment provision. Instead they emphasised the value placed upon social contact.

❖ This point was further emphasised by views about sources of personal support. Those least favoured were psychiatrists and the most favoured were other patients.

❖ Patients preferred voluntary service contact to that with statutory services.

These critical themes brought into question whether psychiatric patients can, in any meaningful sense, be construed as 'consumers'. Being excluded from employment in the main, psychiatric patients are a group with very little 'buying power'. They do not constitute a large market for private practitioners. Contact with services for those with mental health problems is far more extensive than for most others who use health and social services. Psychiatric patients often spend many years of their lives in contact with services and professionals.

The consequences of being labelled 'ill' are serious for a person who is given a psychiatric diagnosis. Since the diagnosis of a person as 'mentally ill' is done primarily on the basis of a judgment about a person's conduct, there is always a risk of invalidating their whole identity or sense of self. Those labelled as mentally ill are discriminated against by present and prospective employers and, as a result, are often subjected to a life of poverty. Educational opportunities are curtailed, family and intimate relationships affected and making social contact with people is fraught with difficulties (Sayce, 2000).

Against this background of social exclusion, satisfaction research about mental health services has commonly adopted a needs assessment approach, which has been less than sensitive to the patient's wider social context and total experience of life. It has usually assessed patient satisfaction according to 'normative need' (defined by current social norms) or 'defined need' (what professionals consider the patient needs). When defining need and casting expressed need about the patient's total life experience into doubt, professionals (maybe with a wry smile) distinguish between what patients 'want' and what they 'need'. 'Wants' are readily connoted as irrational or even frivolous. Paternalism is thus reproduced in a new guise. The assessment of 'insight' is central to this distinction between the patient's view and that of others (Carter, 2003).

There is a small amount of research conducted which does not presume that the professional view of need is self-evidently superior. Rather than 'normative' or 'defined' need this research has focused on 'felt' or 'expressed' need. 'Felt need' is an unexpressed experiential state of wanting something. If articulated it is 'expressed need'. 'Felt need' can be elicited during research or audit exercises. An early example of this was Mayer and Timms' (1970) work in which social workers were encouraged to take seriously the views expressed by clients. The work of Beresford and Croft (1986) also highlights the views of users of social services and emphasises the need for genuine participation by users in research about services.

Whilst professionally defined needs tend to focus on behaviour and the effectiveness of prescribed treatments, 'felt need' evaluations tend to emphasise the material and social aspects of people's everyday lives. Kay and Legg (1986) found that the need to have a job was a high priority for those recently discharged from hospital. Another example is a survey which examined the expressed needs of patients, vis-à-vis their living arrangements and material and social support (Hatfield et al., 1992). A sizeable minority of patients expressed dissatisfaction with their living arrangements. Those living in staffed accom- modation were particularly critical and did not view their living situations as a result of their own positive choice.

Another survey of discharged patients revealed a number of aspects about their qual- ity of life in the community. These included their sense of vulnerability, the benefits of community care, an appreciation of the support of others, an awareness of the impact of scarce resources and disappointment about poor co-ordination between health and social services (MacDonald & Sheldon, 1997). Similarly the vulnerable identity of psy- chiatric patients living in the community has been documented by Barham and Hayward (1991).

The quality assurance literature reflects the way in which the psychiatric patient's voice has been co-opted. However, there are logical and political problems in simply utilising this voice as 'consumer feedback', analogous to hotel guests completing satisfaction questionnaires. The two greatest impediments to this sort of aspiration (held by optimis- tic politicians and service managers) are the enduring social control role of mental health services and the powerful inertia of a bio-medical approach to care. Together they lead to de-humanising outcomes and are at odds with the current policy rhetoric of consumerism and 'patient-centredness'.

A confluence of interests reproduces these impediments. The anxieties of the sane (vot- ing) majority and the prejudice this creates in their minds are important. Politicians and the mass media reflect and reinforce this bias in the public mentality. In the public domain, there remains a preoccupation with the need to control madness. For its part, the psychiatric profession is still dominated by a bio-medical viewpoint, reflected in its retention of the importance of diagnosis and its preference for pharmacological fixes to 'madness' and misery.

These two pillars of orthodoxy – the imperative to control mentally disordered conduct and its treatment within a bio-medical paradigm – may have been moderately shaken by user involvement but they have certainly not been removed. Indeed the emergence of the users' movement and user involvement coincided with the 'decade of the brain' and the triumphalism it spawned in biological psychiatrists (Guze, 1989).

Conclusion

The mental health service user movement, like other new social movements, has asserted a collective voice based upon a shared experience (of mental health problems and mental health services). It has been shouted on the streets and rehearsed in small, smoky settings. It has been driven primarily by anger and frustration, not the desire to aid the smooth running and credibility of local mental health services.

Arguably this hostility has been overly focused on the psychiatric profession. A more even-handed analysis reveals a much wider devaluation of the mad experience in society.

Indeed, the psychiatric profession has increasingly been at pains to encourage public tolerance about mental abnormality. The recent campaign of the Royal College of Psychiatrists, Changing Minds, emphasises the random affliction of mental illness – one in four people affected during their life span (see www.rcpsych.ac.uk/campaigns/cminds). It could be me. It could be you. The logic goes that this roulette randomness demands that we de-stigmatise mental illness and accept and treat it like any other.

A critical response to this campaign might point out that it may be one in four but not any one in four; some social groups are much more prone to mental health problems than others (Rogers & Pilgrim, 2003). Also mental illness is not like physical illness (no matter how much many psychiatrists and some others would like it to be). Its conceptual validity and aetiology [cause] are constantly contested and queried. Patients often do not embrace the diagnosis offered to them because it adds to their demoralisation and stigma. Other illnesses do not regularly warrant the legal deprivation of liberty without trial.

This recent campaign to de-stigmatise mental illness is implicitly bound up with a long term professionalising strategy to make psychiatry a medical specialty like any other. In the 19th century this began with medicine asserting (with no evidence) that madness was a brain disease. In the 1970s the strategy was linked to the shift from the asylum to the District General Hospital, where psychiatry became another proper medical department among many (Baruch & Treacher, 1977). Today the strategy extends to making mental illness one like any other.

But the dominant threads of oppression identified by the users' movement remain. The biomedical model in psychiatry still predominates. The assertion that madness is a brain disease (with little more evidence) is still a professional orthodoxy. The right to diagnose and treat are still privileged over the patient's right to be left alone.

Within the users' movement, all voices are listened to because the libertarianism typical of new social movements tolerates and encourages difference. One wing of this range has eschewed services and co-option, emphasising instead an oppositional agenda including: the abolition of psychiatry; an emphasis on self-help and user-led services; and the end of coercion. On the other wing, the reformist position, with the support of 'professional allies', has offered itself up for co-option under the terms and conditions of user involvement in local services. The offer has been encouraged by the national and local state.

Whereas the voice of protest has been *asserted,* the voice of consumerism has been *elicited*. The British State, under all governments since 1979, has encouraged consumerism in its health and welfare reforms. What we have witnessed in the last 20 years is a limit-testing exercise in user involvement, prompted by this political philosophy (Bowl, 1996;

Barnes & Shardlow, 1997; Bhui *et al.,* 1998; Pilgrim & Waldron, 1998; Truman & Raine, 2002; Diamond *et al.*, 2003; Rose, 2003; Rutter *et al.*, 2004).

User involvement endorses the voice of the patient. It is entreated and attended to, but on terms strictly circumscribed by those controlling the service status quo: managers and professionals. It is in the gift of the latter powerful groups to issue this invitation more or less enthusiastically and with more or less good faith. The existence of mental health services, mental health professionals and their preferred methods of interventions are taken as givens. Professionals and managers may listen to all viewpoints. They may concede feedback and genuinely seek to change services. But they always do so from a position of power. Whereas the users' movement could countenance a world without mental health services, user involvement assumes that they are here to stay. They are only reformable in a way that potentially suits all parties, including those currently at the helm.

The role being demanded of professionals and services from central government, with a mandate from the sane majority, has shifted towards a greater emphasis on risk mini-misation and thus on conservative decision making, which encourages greater levels of coercive control. This shift was reinforced by large hospital closure, leaving smaller, over-stretched acute units prioritising the most risky cases. User involvement and other state-encouraged initiatives (such as advocacy) are retained as mitigating policies, in the midst of this larger shift towards a widening state apparatus to suppress deviance (as in the current Draft Mental Health Bill). This shift has inevitably constrained the achievable aspirations of user involvement.

Finally, there is another position which should be flagged for completeness. Prior to the users' movement, with its identity politics, and managerialism, with its sweeping bow to consumerism, there was an extensive piece of mental health work, which continues to exist: psychotherapy. From the point at which asylum doctors for a short while fell out of favour with government after the First World War (Stone, 1985) to the present, psychotherapists have claimed special expertise in eliciting and formulating the meaning of personal accounts.

Psychotherapy has certainly offered itself as a more humane alternative to drugs, electric-ity and the scalpel but it has retained an individualistic ideology, constructing atomised individual case studies with its clients. Occasionally it has extended this range of case studies of individuals to work on small and large groups. Very occasionally, it has made claims of social insight.

However, this confluence of psychoanalysis and social radicalism has been riven with controversy, with psychoanalysts being reluctant to endorse political excess in their ranks. Despite this factionalism within psychoanalysis, its resonances have been evident in the users' movement. For example, anti-psychiatric spurs for confidence in the users' movement have included the work of Ronald Laing and Thomas Szasz (both psychiatrists and psychoanalysts).

The great bulk of psychotherapy has joined the mental health industry in an adaptive rather than challenging way – particularly in the USA. One of the weaknesses, even of socially radical psychoanalysis, is its overwhelming focus on common mental illness – a reflection of Freud's pessimism about the psychoanalytical treatment of madness. Only a few, such as Laing, took the risk of exploring the latter experience and they were kept firmly on the professional margins or even cast beyond the pale. The reclamation of meaning from madness, which Laing championed, has strong resonances now in the Hearing Voices Network, itself prompted by another psychiatrist, Marius Romme (Romme & Escher, 1993).

For some, psychoanalysis and other forms of psychotherapeutic expertise may retain a mandate to represent the collective voice of mental abnormality. But, in recent times, the service users' movement and consumerism in social policy have underpinned the legitimacy of the patient perspective. For now, they have pushed the psychotherapeutic claim into third place.

2 New Services for Old
– An overview of mental health policy

Jed Boardman

Introduction

When the Sainsbury Centre for Mental Health (SCMH) was created in 1985 as the National Unit for Psychiatric Research and Development, mental health policy and the development of services were at a pivotal point. The closing two decades of the 20th century marked a shift from reforming zeal to a more fragmented pragmatism.

This chapter aims to give an overview of mental health policy in the United Kingdom over the past 20 years and to note some of the key changes that have taken place. But to do this justice we need to examine the policy developments in the preceding decade of the 20th century, and particularly the effects of the developing welfare state after 1948.

Developments before 1948

The development of psychiatric services (later mental health services) during the 20th century has been characterised by a movement away from large mental hospitals, which had grown during the nineteenth century, towards extramural forms of care. This movement was not new and had begun in the nineteenth century when, for example, attempts were made to stimulate an integration of psychiatry into the universities (Hill, 1969). In the early 20th century isolated attempts had been made to establish outpatient departments in general hospitals and there were calls for moves to prevent mental disorder and to provide treatments for those patients with disorders not severe enough to warrant incarceration. In 1923 these aims were realised, to some degree, when the Maudsley Hospital was opened to provide treatment for 'voluntary' (informal) patients.

The 1930 Mental Treatment Act was the first official Act since the 1890 Lunacy Act to be directly concerned with the mentally ill. It introduced the possibility of informal admission to mental hospitals, emphasised the importance of community support and aftercare, and encouraged the development of outpatient departments and the opening of observation wards. However, in practice little changed and the practice of psychiatry remained firmly in the large asylums, headed by the medical superintendents and administered by the local authorities.

Developments 1948-1970

The National Health Service (NHS) came into being on 5 July 1948 and with it came the beginning of the development of the modern welfare state that provided the conditions for a shift in policy and practice (Rose, 2001). The provision of social welfare benefits meant that it was no longer necessary to remove the unwaged mentally ill to asylums, and the provision of public housing meant that they could be sheltered outside institutions. In addition, the development of an improved system of primary medical care allowed general practitioners to provide drug treatments in non-custodial settings, and the consolidation of medical and psychiatric social work within local authorities allowed for supervision outside hospitals.

The NHS inherited a large number of municipal, voluntary and mental hospitals which were nationalised and, importantly for psychiatry, meant that mental hospitals operated under the same conditions as other branches of medicine. But the mental hospitals still had a separate governance system, under the Lunacy and Mental Treatment Acts, which required that the Chief Officer should be the Medical Superintendent.

By the 1950s the need for a change in legislation became increasingly apparent and was met by the 1959 Mental Health Act. This new legislation was an outcome of the Royal Commission on Mental Illness and Mental Deficiency, 1954-1957. The Commission had been set up for several reasons (Ramon, 1982). First, the 1930 Act had not repealed the 1890 Act, making legislation too cumbersome. Second, the general atmosphere of affluence encouraged contemplation of further, more liberal, legislation. Third, the media, MPs and professionals were pressing for changes as a result of a series of scandals and concern about poor hospital conditions. Finally, the burden on services, both inpatient and outpatient, was increasing.

The intent of the 1959 Act was "to repeal the Lunacy and Mental Treatments Acts, 1890 to 1930, and the Mental Deficiency Acts, 1913 to 1938 and to make fresh provision with respect to the treatment of mentally disordered persons and with respect to their property and affairs" (quoted in Rollin, 1977). The Act emphasised community care (indeed the Royal Commission's report was the first government publication to use this term) and implicitly obliged the community (in the form of the local authority) to set up services for those who did not need or no longer needed inpatient care. However, as with the 1930 Act, this was not mandatory and there was no date set for meeting the recommendation of the Royal Commission that central government should provide direct financial support to local authorities for community care.

The occupancy of beds in mental hospitals reached a peak in 1955, after which it began to decline. During the early 1960s optimistic forecasts were produced concerning the reduction of beds in mental hospitals. These were seized upon by the Minister of Health, Enoch Powell, and in 1962 the Conservative Government produced a *Hospital Plan for England and Wales* (Ministry of Health, 1962). A year later they produced *Health and Welfare: The Development of Community Care* (Ministry of Health, 1963). These set the scene for future government policy and predicted that by 1975 there would be a reduction by nearly half in the numbers of local hospital beds and that there would be a split between community agencies and general hospitals.

The development of alternatives to the large mental hospitals began, but was slow and patchy, often relying on enthusiastic and dedicated innovators. Psychiatric units were developed in District General Hospitals, beginning in the Manchester area. Outpatient departments opened; the beginnings of a community psychiatric nursing service emerged; day hospitals were established. But there was no effective system of planning, no overall organisation of community services and no financial backing to allow substantial development. Warnings were made at an early stage that community care for the mentally ill was not helpful if the rhetoric could not be met with adequate resources (Titmuss, 1961).

In the early 1970s, the reorganisation of welfare services by the integration of social work into the new local authority social services departments, recommended in the document known as the Seebohm Report (Barratt *et al.*, 1968), removed the psychiatric social workers from their otherwise collaborative roles with mental health services.

The context in which this post-war development of psychiatry occurred was that of the Keynesian Welfare State. The optimism and hope generated in this period brought with it three major developments in the care of people with mental health problems: the open door policy; the introduction of antipsychotic and antidepressant medication in the 1950s; and the drive to put care back into the community at large (Jones, 1972). Added to these were the desire for psychiatry to gain the status of other medical specialities, and the costs of incarceration and the maintenance of buildings (Rose, 2001). The move away from asylums was supported by research findings demonstrating the importance of living conditions on elements of behaviour and symptom formation previously accepted as an inherent characteristic of the disease itself (e.g. Wing & Brown, 1970).

The impetus to empty asylums existed prior to the development of the new drugs – studies in Britain and elsewhere in Europe had revealed that the introduction of new drugs made only modest impacts on release figures (Shepherd *et al.*, 1961; Odegard, 1964). Later claims that discharge and the re-emergence of social rehabilitation were due largely to the introduction of effective medical treatments are not substantiated by the evidence. Increased discharge rates, shorter stays in hospital and day care for chronic patients were accepted norms in advanced centres before the introduction of effective new medications. Nonetheless, drug therapy did play an important role and fuelled optimism. As a result, more patients than hitherto became candidates for open wards, and later for placement in the community.

Within this post-war era of corporatist politics grew a number of influential anti-psychiatry movements. These emphasised the mirage of diagnostic categories (e.g. Szasz, 1961), the dangers of hospitals (e.g. Rosenham, 1973), the role of society and the family as primary causal factors in mental illness (e.g. Bateson, 1972; Laing & Esterson, 1964) and the meaningfulness of psychotic phenomena, such as delusions (Laing, 1960). These provided a radical perspective on the need for deinstitutionalisation.

The 1970s

The year 1971 witnessed the first clear statement of government policy *Hospital Services for the Mentally Ill* (DHSS, 1971) which emphasised the importance of non-hospital facilities, and the gradual phasing out of large mental hospitals and their replacement by District General Hospital (DGH) units. In 1975 the White Paper *Better Services for the Mentally Ill* (DHSS, 1975) attempted to provide an analysis of objectives and means of making progress towards a new pattern of services based on experience since 1962. It set out four broad policy objectives, as shown in Box 1.

Box 1: The policy objectives of the 1975 White Paper *Better Services for the Mentally Ill*

1. Expansion of local authority residential, day care and social work support services.

2. Relocation of specialist services in local settings.

3. Establishment of the correct organisational links between day and residential care services, between specialist teams and primary care services, between local authority administrators and planners and between professionals and non-professionals.

4. Staffing improvements which would make possible assessment, review, early intervention and preventative work.

The White Paper emphasised that the suggested guidelines were tentative and that "...even in favourable economic circumstances it would obviously take a long-term programme to achieve in all parts of the country the kind of change we are advocating...even within a 25 year planning horizon...discharge from a hospital into a community which lacks the hospital facilities...may well be a change for the worse".

If the building blocks of the services had been put down in the 1950s and 1960s, then the 1970s were a time of modest expansion. Rates of bed occupancy fell from a maximum of 350 per 100,000 population in 1954 to 151 per 100,000 in 1982. In general, overall admission rates increased owing to the increase in readmissions, but the number of new admissions fell until the 1970s. There was an associated decrease in the length of admissions and an increase in the proportion of elderly residents. By 1975 there were 130 psychiatric units in DGHs and this figure rose to 164 by 1981.

The day care of patients was a typically British concern and the first day hospital was established by Josuah Bierer in 1946. The number of day hospitals increased from two in 1949 to 65 in 1966. By 1975 there were 6,000 day hospital places and this rose to 15,300 by 1981. Day centres, meanwhile, were created by local authorities and the first one opened in 1945, but it was not until the creation of local authority Social Service Departments in 1971 that they showed significant development. The number of day centre places rose from 3,403 in 1975 to 5,025 in 1982. The number of places in homes and hostels rose from 3,911 in 1975 to 6,044 in 1981, the main increase being in unstaffed accommodation.

The 1980s onwards

The context has now been set for the examination of the changes in policy and services since 1985. The basis of the modern mental health service had already been laid, but no asylum had yet been closed and only a few community mental health teams and centres existed (the first were set up in 1978) (Sayce et al., 1991). Mental health services were under-funded and the main resources were locked in the large hospitals. By the end of the 1970s the political and social climate had changed.

Since the mid 1970s two identifiable transformations had occurred in the core capitalist states: a general shift to the right of many governments and a decline in the economic climate. The transformations represented a crisis of capital occurring in several economic, political and ideological dimensions. In economic terms the symptoms of the crisis included high levels of unemployment and inflation, a reduction in output and world trade and a growth in the public debt. In political and ideological terms it was represented by a rolling back of the boundaries of the state and an emphasis on the values of individualism. In the UK this was represented by the policies of 'Thatcherism': a social market economy and 'authoritarian populism' (Hall & Jacques, 1983). These changes were to have an effect on health services in general and mental health policies in particular.

When SCMH opened in 1985, there were two government documents that highlighted the concerns and changes for the 1980s. In 1983 the new Mental Health Act came into operation. This was a consolidation of the 1959 Act and the Mental Health (Amendment) Act, 1982. Its main emphasis was on patients' rights and it was criticised for the introduction of legalism and bureaucracy – factors that would influence policy in the next two decades. Like the 1959 Act it made recommendations about patient care but the only legal obligation was for local authorities to provide aftercare facilities for some compulsorily detained patients.

No new resources were allocated to meet the provisions of the 1983 Act. This inadequacy of funding was acknowledged by the report of the House of Commons Social Services Committee (DHSS, 1985) which had received evidence from health services, professional and voluntary bodies and concluded that they were "providing a mental disability service which is under-financed and under-staffed both in its health and social service aspects". It made three important recommendations regarding health service fiscal policy. First, that policy could only be achieved by a real increase in expenditure; second, that an equivalent proportion of the resources, services and amenities devoted to the most severely mentally disabled should continue to be so devoted in the future; third, that the DHSS should create a central bridging fund. This final recommendation was to figure highly in debates about how to create feasible community services so that the large institutions might be closed.

Two years before the opening of the Sainsbury Centre for Mental Health, the Department of Health had issued a directive to Regional Health Authorities requiring them to attempt to close their large psychiatric institutions. But the NHS faced a critical Catch 22. They had to close institutions whilst at the same time creating effective community services that were adequately financed at the time when all health and social services were under-funded. This led to a series of documents highlighting the plight of patients in the community (e.g. Audit Commission, 1986; 1992; 1994), policy being increasingly directed towards those with severe mental illness (Care Programme Approach, Supervision Registers, Ten Point Plan) and the introduction of the NHS internal market (Griffiths, 1988; *NHS and Community Care Act*, House of Commons, 1990)

During the past 20 years one component has been significant: the increase in official government and voluntary sector documents relating to mental health policy. Prior to the 1980s such documents were uncommon and the majority have been covered earlier in this chapter, but the past 20 years have seen repeated moves to re-organise NHS services and an increasing concern about the provision of services. A brief survey of the Department of Health website (www.dh.gov.uk) at the end of 2004 revealed over 60 official publications directly relating to mental health policy in England. In view of this it is not feasible to review all official policy documents and their development, so the remainder of this chapter will examine main trends in policy over the past 20 years.

Managing risk

Perhaps the most profound change in policy since the 1970s has been related to mechanisms for the control of risk. This is reflected in the types of services that have developed and in the obligations of mental health workers and the organisations providing care. With the demise of the asylums control of patients living in the community has been of central concern. Whereas before the high profile incidents that led to official inquiries related to poor practice and care (e.g. DHSS, 1969) in recent years it has been highly visible tragedies involving the public and others (e.g. DHSS, 1988; Ritchie *et al.*, 1994) that have precipitated policy change.

In common with the rest of the NHS since the 1984 Griffiths Report (Griffiths, 1984), policymakers have sought increasingly bureaucratised solutions such as the Care Programme Approach and the introduction of supervision registers. The new assertive outreach services are an attempt to form highly organised supervision teams for people whose behaviour is regarded as problematic and hard to engage. The increase in the number of medium secure units offers another institutional solution to mental illness and contributes to the return to asylums along with the virtual asylums of hostels and homes for the mentally ill.

The state has been accused of increasing the social control functions of mental health professions, most notably in its attempts to bring in a new Mental Health Act, which has been vigorously opposed by an alliance of mental health professionals, voluntary and charitable organisations and the legal profession. Dubious official pronouncements that 'community care has failed' have been voiced, often as a prelude to further policy developments of control.

Current policy and trends

During the 1990s mental health attained a higher profile and priority among government policies, reflected perhaps by its inclusion as one of the priority areas in the 1993 *Health of the Nation* White Paper (DH, 1992) which set out key priority areas for health in England and Wales. It has retained this status and the first of the Labour government's National Service Frameworks (NSFs) was for Mental Health in adults of working age (DH, 1999). Subsequent NSFs have included mental health care for children (DH, 2004c) and for adults over 65 years (DH, 2001). The Mental Health NSF has been generally welcomed but has been criticised for its prescriptive nature. It has added to the range of services for people with mental health problems and has highlighted the need for improved mental health promotion and the provision of services in primary care. The NSFs have been brought in with the associated promise of increased spending on the health service as a whole and mental health services in particular, but the increased funding may not have been getting down to the local services (SCMH, 2003).

Standards in mental health services still fall below the rest of the NHS despite the clear advances in treatment and provision of services over the past 20 years: for example Mental Health Trusts were more likely than Acute Trusts to receive a zero star rating in recent assessments (Healthcare Commission, 2004). Increases in funding have been required throughout the post-war period and it remains a concern that funding remains low and poorly distributed (DH, 2004a). Some areas such as mental health promotion, primary care services and rehabilitation remain poorly developed (possibly as a consequence of the focus on acute care associated with the emphasis on control).

The true costs of the Mental Health NSF are probably not realised and are likely to be far greater than the increases in funding have allowed for, and there is certainly a shortfall of trained staff to deliver its demands (DH, 2004b). The commissioning of services is also poorly developed. The effectiveness of the chosen approach of using targets and inspections to improve quality remains to be seen.

Across medicine there has been an increasing demand for evidence-based treatments, represented at the policy level by the creation of the National Institute for Clinical Excellence (NICE), and this as a whole has been well received in mental health practice, perhaps because of the recognition that many historical practices have had dubious validity. Nevertheless, the evidence base in mental health service provision is weak, despite improvements in research over the past two decades, and an exclusive reliance on scientific forms of knowledge has been questioned (Laugharne, 2004).

The changing demographics of society and increasing geographical mobility have altered the social environment in which mental health services are delivered. Policies have now been issued with regard to ethnicity and social exclusion (e.g. DH, 2005; SEU, 2004). A dominant response to changing societal demands has been to place the idea of choice into service policy. This may reflect no more than populist government policies. It indicates the consumerist stance of policy making and indeed may be of little relevance to many with severe mental illness. At its best it reflects an important change towards the increasing voice of users in public services (DH, 2000).

There has been a welcome and increasing emphasis on the central position of the patient or user in the delivery and planning of public services. The previous hegemony of the professions has to a significant extent been eroded away. For health care professionals as a whole, and mental health professionals in particular, these moves create their own tensions. Health care is a competitive economy and not only are professionals asked to provide expert opinions and clear communication that resonates with users' wishes, but they are also expected to act as gatekeepers to finite resources acting on professional judgements not patient preference. This is a political nettle that has yet to be grasped: a policy based around the voice of the consumer, with its associated rising expectations, cannot be met at the same time as resources are restricted. For mental health professionals, demands for increasing social control provide an additional dimension at a time when users are encouraged to demand an increasing say in their treatments and in the practice of services.

The context of mental health policy in the 1990s to some degree reflects the changes begun in the late 1970s with the rolling back of welfare state provision and a move from collectivist ideologies to an increasing emphasis on individuals and a growing reliance on multi-agency and market solutions to the delivery of public services. The crisis of capitalism in the 1970s gave way to a renewed confidence in its dominant ideologies following the demise of Communism in Eastern Europe. Management of the UK economy has allowed increases in public spending, but the move of public service provision as a whole remains in the direction of a mixed economy with ever increasing emphasis on private sector provision (Pollock, 2004).

There remain, however, essential tensions and contradictions at the heart of policy. The gap between rich and poor has increased over recent years and we are facing widening inequalities in society which have implications for the health of both individuals and communities; evidence suggests that what matters within societies is not so much the direct health effects of absolute living standards so much as the effects of social inequalities (Wilkinson, 1996). Health is powerfully affected by social position and by the scale of social and economic differences among the population. In the developed world, it is not the richest countries that have the best health but the most egalitarian. Wilkinson (1996) argues that an important characteristic shared by the healthy egalitarian societies is social cohesion: that they have a strong community life. Thus instead of social life stopping outside the front door, public space remains a social space; individualism and the values of the market are restrained by social morality; people are more likely to be involved in social and voluntary activities outside the home; there are fewer signs of antisocial aggressiveness and society is more caring. In short the social fabric is in better condition.

This is crucial to mental health and illness and is a barrier to improving the mental health of the nation and the social environment in which mental health services are delivered.

Conclusion

Mental health policy has changed over the course of the 20th century as have the location and practice of mental health services. The central shift occurred after the Second World War with the development of the modern welfare state, which provided some of the material and ideological conditions to move from institutional care to community-based services. The post war consensus began to be eroded in the last quarter of the 20th century and the optimism of the post war decades now seems like a bygone age. The shift in policy has been from one that reflected this optimism to one that pays increasing attention to control. Nevertheless, almost 200 years after they began, all the asylums in England have closed, many have been sold, there are an increasing number of community-based facilities, and fears about the ex-inmates of institutions filling the ranks of the homeless have not been realised. And mental health matters have at last become a real priority for health policy, as evidenced in the ever increasing number of policy documents produced on the subject.

Direct threats to mental health services come from their continued under-funding, patchy policy implementation, the continued fragmentation of services, the growing emphasis on social control and the chronic shortfall of trained personnel. Broader threats arise from the increasing inequality seen both at a national and a global level and from the neo-liberal policies which have given rise to it. Modern practice arose from the development of welfare state provision and modern services have been developed on the back of these. Today the very concerns that gave rise to the welfare state sixty years ago are as powerful and as urgent as ever.

3 Acute Care in Crisis

Lesley Warner

Introduction

In 1985, someone looking for help with a mental health problem could expect to be treated in a psychiatric hospital. They could also expect their local hospital to be a former asylum, about a hundred years old, located outside their town or city, consisting of large buildings in extensive grounds and identifiable by a prominent water tower which was visible for miles around. Community-based approaches such as day hospitals and community psychiatric nurses had been in existence since the 1950s, but service provision was patchy and in most areas did not represent a realistic alternative to inpatient care. By 1986, official figures showed that although over 80% of people with mental health problems were living in the community, more than 80% of the available resources were being spent on hospital care (NIMHE, 2003).

In 2005, someone with that same mental health problem could expect a very different approach to be offered by a range of crisis resolution/home treatment teams, crisis houses, partial hospitalisation, early intervention services, assertive outreach teams and multidisciplinary community mental health teams, provided by a combination of health, social care and voluntary sector organisations. This chapter tells the story of the transition from NHS-run institutional care, to the mosaic of residential and community-based services from a range of providers that we have today.

Numbers of beds/hospitals

In 1987/88, the total number of psychiatric beds had fallen from a peak of 154,000 in 1954 to around 67,000 (DH, 2004a). The number of beds has continued to fall, so that by 2003/04, the most recent year for which the information is available, there were 32,400 altogether, of which 13,261 were acute care beds for adults, a further 2,500 were beds in secure units, and the remainder were 'long stay' beds (i.e. non-acute care and beds for people in other age groups) (DH, 2004b).

A number of factors contributed to this reduction in beds. Enoch Powell, as minister of health, started the move towards community care in 1961 by announcing his vision for mental health services over the next 15 years, including a closure and re-provision programme for the 'water tower hospitals' (Powell, 1961). Not underestimating the resistance his plan would encounter, Powell had urged "ruthlessness" in the pursuit of "drastic and fundamental change" in order to improve mental health care. But the closure programme did not really get going until the mid 1970s, following the publication of the White Paper *Better Services for the Mentally Ill* (DHSS, 1975), and the first full hospital closure did not take place until 1986 (Stewart, 2003). The re-provision programme resettled large numbers of former long-stay patients into smaller residential units in the community. It also led to acute psychiatric inpatient units being built on District General Hospital sites, a move that helped to dispel some of the stigma associated with using mental health services. The concept of 'care in the community', shaped by numerous policy and consultation documents, was to become the mantra for mental health services for the next two decades and beyond.

Of the 130 psychiatric hospitals in England and Wales in 1975, 116 have now closed and the others are much reduced in size (Mahoney, 2004). Although this programme is largely complete nationally, some NHS trusts are still finalising plans for new units to replace these large institutions. At the same time, a second wave of re-provision is under way as commissioners and providers of acute inpatient services re-evaluate the suitability of their premises to meet the needs of the 21st century, with a move towards creating smaller, more domestic-style units. Recent central requirements on the provision of single sex accommodation are also affecting the design of new acute inpatient units (NHSE, 2000).

However, recent research suggests that six European countries, including England, have been undergoing a process of reinstitutionalisation during the past decade, based on an increase in the number of forensic beds and places in supported housing (Priebe *et al.*, 2005). It further suggests that a similar increase in the prison population during this period is also contributing to an institutional response to the containment of perceived risk.

The impact of changing policy on acute inpatient services

The theme of mental health policy during the last 20 years has been the growth and development of community-based services alongside a reduction in the reliance on inpatient care. An understanding of some of the key government policies and guidance relating to, or affecting, inpatient care is helpful in seeing how far acute services have come.

Box 1: Policies and guidance affecting acute inpatient care 1975-2002

1975: *Better Services for the Mentally Ill* (DHSS, 1975)
This White Paper set the scene for developments throughout the 1980s and beyond, describing the way in which NHS, local authority and voluntary sector agencies should provide an integrated mental health service, with the focus on community-based services.

1988: *Community Care – agenda for action* (Griffiths, 1988)
The Audit Commission (1986) had reported that although hospitals were reducing in size, community services were not sufficiently resourced to provide alternative types of care. This led to Roy Griffiths' 1988 report, which proposed the transfer of all community care to local authorities.

1989: *Caring for People* (DHSS, 1989)
This White Paper, a response to the Griffiths' report, set out the framework for changes to community care, including a split between the purchasing and providing functions of health and social care agencies, and an encouragement of the use of a broad spectrum of services, including independent as well as statutory sector providers.

1990: *National Health Service and Community Care Act* (House of Commons, 1990)
This gave local authorities responsibility for community care assessments and provision and introduced the Care Programme Approach (CPA), effective from 1991, as the framework for the care for people with mental health problems.

1993: *Health of the Nation, Key Area Handbook, Mental Health* (DH, 1993)
This expanded on the three mental illness targets set out in the 1992 *Health of the Nation*. The targets included significantly improving the health and social functioning of mentally ill people, and reducing suicide rates.

1996: *The Spectrum of Care: Local services for people with mental health problems* (DH, 1996)
This handbook summarised the core components that should make up a comprehensive local service for people with mental health problems. It included information on the types of treatment and the range of settings for treatment and social care, including 24-hour care for people in acute mental health crisis.

1997: *The New NHS: Modern, Dependable* (DH, 1997)
This White Paper included the replacement of the NHS internal market with new funding arrangements, reforming the 'purchaser/provider split' that had begun in 1991.

1998: *A First Class Service: Quality in the New NHS* (DH, 1998a)
This strategy paper announced the intention to set national standards through evidence-based National Service Frameworks, along with the formation of the National Institute for Clinical Excellence (NICE) which would produce guidance on

Box 1: Policies and guidance affecting acute inpatient care 1975-2002 *(continued)*

clinically- and cost-effective treatments. It also set out a number of initiatives to monitor the quality of services provided: clinical governance within health care providers, the formation of the Commission for Health Improvement (CHI), and the establishment of a performance framework.

1998: ***Modernising Mental Health Services: Safe, Sound and Supportive*** (DH, 1998b)
This presented the Government's strategy for reforming mental health services for the adult population and announced a massive injection of funding over three years. In a Foreword, Frank Dobson, the Secretary of State, made the startling statement that "care in the community has failed". The document went on to make a commitment to ensuring there were "enough beds of the right kind in the right place", stating that in some areas, particularly London, there would need to be more beds for acute care.

1999: ***National Service Framework (NSF) for Mental Health*** (DH, 1999)
This set national standards for mental health services, mostly focused on elements of community services. Standard five says that people who need "a period of care away from their home" should have timely access to a hospital bed, or an alternative place, in the least restrictive environment and as close to home as possible.

2000: ***The NHS Plan*** (DH, 2000)
Most of the focus of this 10-year plan was on community-based services such as the development of a range of specialist teams. While part of the rationale of the new services was to reduce pressure on beds, the *NHS Plan* gave no specific mention to acute mental health hospitals at all.

2001: ***The Mental Health Policy Implementation Guide*** (DH, 2001)
This supported the delivery of adult mental health policy at the local level, following on from the *NHS Plan* and the *NSF*. Although emphasising the need to see mental health services as "whole systems", it too did not address acute inpatient services, merely acknowledging their importance and promising guidance at a later date.

2002: ***Mental Health Policy Implementation Guide: Adult Acute Inpatient Provision*** (DH, 2002)
This describes acute inpatient care as "a core and integral component of the *NSF* to which all the *NSF* standards are relevant", making the point that despite the reduction in bed numbers, more is spent annually on hospitals than on community services. It provided guidance on how to improve services, acknowledging the importance of the physical, psychological and therapeutic environments of care. It said inpatient care was one possible response – rather than the only option – to someone needing care at a time of mental health crisis.

The therapeutic inpatient environment

Those who commission services increasingly expect to be able to draw on published research evidence to help shape their view of what they should fund. In this evidence-based climate, it is instructive to be reminded of Muijen's warning (2002) that there remains no research evidence demonstrating "the therapeutic effectiveness of hospital care as compared with other services". He adds that the key to therapeutic care is investing in inpatient staff – their recruitment, training and retention – and in designing services "around the wishes of the patient", without which wards will "neither be therapeutic nor safe". Yet in the late 1990s and early 2000s, a number of research studies looked at what was happening in acute inpatient units, and found many causes for concern.

In 1998, the Sainsbury Centre for Mental Health examined inpatient care in 38 sites across the country, focusing in more depth on a representative sample of nine inpatient wards and interviewing 112 inpatients (SCMH, 1998). This study found that one in ten people had been admitted for the 'wrong' reasons – social reasons or respite care. Nearly three-quarters of all patients who were on the wards two months later probably did not need to be there. Serious deficiencies in the standard of care offered by acute inpatient services were identified. In particular, the care provided did not meet individuals' social and therapeutic needs, the ward environment was generally poor and lacking in amenities, and the needs of specific groups of patients were not separately addressed.

One of the most striking findings, common to a number of studies (including those by Barker, 2000, and McGeorge & Lindow, 2000), is that inpatients often feel unsafe in hospital, with some experiencing harassment and verbal or physical abuse. Mind's current 'Ward Watch' campaign (2004) is backed by a survey that found many respondents still felt unsafe in hospital, that mixed sex wards were still common, that patients felt they were not helped by being in hospital and that patients were not treated with respect by staff.

One service user's chronicle of life on a psychiatric ward, (Antoniou, 2000) highlighted another common problem – the boredom and frustration of the inpatient routine. This was echoed by a number of service users who reported that boredom was the most consistent feature of their inpatient stays (Rose, 2001).

The role of service users in monitoring standards in acute services has increased over the past decade through initiatives such as User-Focused Monitoring (UFM). Many hospitals have undergone this process, in which groups of users design, co-ordinate and implement reviews of services and make recommendations for improvement. This approach is currently being used in at least 10 NHS trusts across the country.

An attempt at making things better in acute care is currently being undertaken by four English trusts that are trying to develop new ways of providing acute inpatient care, keeping service users at the heart of the process, through participating in SCMH's *The*

Search for Acute Solutions project. This three year project aims to improve life on the wards through local programmes of staff development and training and through service development.

Monitoring acute inpatient care

The Commission for Health Improvement (CHI) was established to monitor the quality of care provided by NHS Trusts. Through regular clinical governance visits to inpatient units, CHI built up a picture of life in mental health acute inpatient units, publishing a digest of their findings in *What CHI has found in mental health trusts* (2003). The report revealed high bed occupancy rates, of over 150% in some places. The Healthcare Commission has now taken over the role of monitoring health care provision from CHI, and is expected to continue with a similar monitoring programme, at least in the short term.

The Mental Health Act Commission (MHAC) is a special health authority with a statutory remit to monitor the operation of the Mental Health Act 1983 in respect of detained patients. It carries out a regular visiting programme to review the operation of the Act in mental health hospitals, which includes inspecting records and interviewing detained patients. 'Count Me In', the first national census of all inpatients in England and Wales, on 31 March 2005, is being led by the MHAC in collaboration with the National Institute for Mental Health in England (NIMHE) and the Healthcare Commission (MHAC, 2004).

The physical environment

The Royal College of Psychiatrists has contributed to the thinking on the constituents of an ideal acute inpatient unit through their working party report on "the size, staffing, siting and structure of new acute adult psychiatric inpatient units" (RCP, 1998). They recommended setting up project teams involving clinicians, service users, carers, and the voluntary sector to plan new units and their operational policies. They felt that the ideal unit's size would be between 10 and 15 beds per ward, consisting of between 3 and 5 wards, no more than two storeys high, and sited on a District General Hospital campus in a convenient location for the population served. They also stressed the importance of high quality design and finish, having a safe area for exercise, ensuring that all sleeping accommodation is in single rooms with en suite facilities, and that women-only communal rooms are provided. Overall, security issues should be an integral part of the design, supported by effective policies and adequate staffing levels, to ensure that wards are – and feel – safe places both for service users and for staff.

Other research studies and reports have identified the role played by the physical environment in the mental health and safety of staff and inpatients alike. An inquiry report by Blom-Cooper *et al.* (1995) found that an inpatient building's unsuitability for its purpose had contributed to a tragic homicide. Other researchers, including Lawson and Phiri (1999, 2000) have highlighted the beneficial effects of a new psychiatric unit compared to the hospital it replaced; in particular, reduced lengths of stay were attributed to the building's improved design.

More recently, the *Health Service Journal* (2004) has been campaigning to improve the physical fabric of mental health units, having identified many wards in sore need of improvement.

Detained patients

Legal provision exists to compel some individuals, who do not accept the need for mental health intervention, to have their mental state assessed and to be treated against their will. The Mental Health Act of 1983 was effectively a re-drafting of the previous Act of 1959, formulated on the basis that hospitals were the keystone of mental health services and that patients subject to the Act would be compulsorily admitted to hospital as a first step towards assessment and treatment. The new Mental Health Bill, currently progressing through the legislative process, changes this assumption by including compulsory orders which can be applied to people living in their own homes.

Department of Health records show that the number of formal admissions to hospital under the Mental Health Act 1983 almost doubled since the end of the 1980s. There were 16,000 formal admissions in 1988-89, rising to a peak of 26,900 in 1998-99, with the most recent figures showing there were 26,700 formal admissions in 2002-03, representing a small increase on the previous year (DH, 2004c).

It has been argued that this increase is related to the proliferation and success of crisis resolution and home treatment teams at keeping out of hospital some people who would in the past have been admitted. While these teams have reduced the overall number of admissions in some areas, the individuals who *are* admitted tend to be those experiencing the most severe mental health problems, who are unable or unwilling to engage with community services, and so are more likely to be compulsorily detained.

The overall decrease in the number of beds may also be a factor, as if only the most acutely ill people can get admitted this may provide a perverse incentive to the staff involved in the process of 'sectioning' to opt for a compulsory admission. In addition, Laurance (2002) argues that the published recommendations of inquiry panels following homicides committed by individuals known to mental health services have contributed to the development in some areas of risk-averse practice, with some clinicians responding to the public's and politicians' fears by an increased use of the Act.

As conditions for inpatients got worse, the situation of those detained against their will also gave cause for concern. In 1996, the Mental Health Act Commission in collaboration with the Sainsbury Centre for Mental Health undertook a 'National Visit' – a one day census in around 47% of all acute mental health inpatient units in England and Wales, looking at issues of bed occupancy, staffing levels, and services for women patients (SCMH, 1997). High bed occupancy rates and low levels of staffing were found, little interaction took place between nurses and patients, and there was a lack of safe facilities for women patients.

A second 'National Visit' in 1999 focused on the care of detained patients from Black and minority ethnic groups (Warner *et al.*, 2000). It examined the recording and monitoring of patients' ethnicity, how racial harassment of patients by other patients and by staff was dealt with, staff access to training in race equality and anti-discriminatory practice, and the provision of, access to, and use of interpreters. It was found that many people from Black and minority ethnic groups were not receiving care that met their cultural, religious and communication needs. Although policies to guide practice in the key areas of recording and monitoring ethnicity, dealing with racial harassment, staff training, and the use of interpreters were not universally in place, some excellent examples of good work were identified.

Workforce issues

Since 1985, staff in acute inpatient units have become the poor relations in a Cinderella service. The new crisis resolution and other new community teams have encouraged experienced clinical staff, mainly nurses, to move out of hospitals into services where they enjoy working in new ways, with more autonomy, and often with higher salaries. This has left many acute inpatient wards denuded of their most experienced staff. Trusts, forced to focus on introducing the new teams, may have had no money to spare for developing their inpatient staff through ongoing training, which has resulted, in some areas, in relatively unskilled, inexperienced and demoralised staff being left on the wards.

There is evidence, however, that acute inpatient staff are once more becoming seen as crucial to providing effective care in all parts of the service. This started with the publication of *The Capable Practitioner* (SCMH, 2001), outlining a unifying framework which encompasses the skills, knowledge and attitudes required within the workforce to effectively implement the National Service Framework for Mental Health, focusing on the key professional disciplines of psychiatry, nursing, occupational therapy, social work, clinical psychology and non-professionally aligned support work. These capabilities were formalised by the Department of Health, through SCMH, in setting out *The Ten Essential Shared Capabilities* that all qualified and non-qualified mental health staff working in the NHS, social care, voluntary and independent sectors, should acquire as part of their core training (NIMHE, 2004).

The training of acute inpatient staff has now been informed by new training guidance (Clarke, 2004) which aims to make current training and development opportunities more relevant and available to inpatient practitioners from all professional groups.

New ways of organising services and configuring teams have presented a challenge to traditional ways of working, and psychiatrists in particular have had to rethink their role as head of the multidisciplinary team. Kennedy and Griffiths (2001), and Colgan (2002) report that some psychiatrists have already changed the way they work, becoming more focused on community-based work or making acute inpatient care a speciality in its own right. Psychiatrists' roles are also coming under national scrutiny, with a multi-agency steering group providing guidance to Trusts, consultant psychiatrists and other professionals on issues such as medical responsibility and new models in order to promote flexibility for local practice to address shortages in psychiatrists and the need to work differently (NIMHE/CWP/RCP/DH, 2004).

Alternatives to inpatient care

Increasingly during the past two decades, acute inpatient hospitals were being seen as just one possible response to people experiencing a mental health crisis, rather than the only option. The growth of crisis resolution/home treatment teams in England during the 1990s and 2000s developed from a model already being used elsewhere. They provided a community-based approach through which many service users were able to remain in their own homes during a period of mental health crisis. Authors who have documented these developments include Stein and Test (1980), Hoult *et al.* (1983) and Johnson and Thornicroft (1991). An evaluation of a pioneering home treatment team in Birmingham concluded that it had reduced inpatient bed usage, increased people's contact with community mental health services, and overall had cost less than a more conventional model of care (Minghella *et al.*, 1998).

Orme and Hogan (2000) report that the role of the voluntary sector in providing care and respite to people in mental health crisis, some provided by service user-led or user-run organisations, was slowly growing in the 1990s. A number of projects were funded in 1996 by the Mental Health Foundation, including residential services, safe houses and telephone support services. An evaluation of some of these services (MHF/SCMH, 2002) concluded that they had an important part to play in the overall range of care for people in a crisis.

Conclusion

To reflect on the position of acute inpatient care at the start of the 21st century, the key to understanding life on acute wards is the expectation that they will fulfil a number of clearly defined roles and functions. Despite Department of Health guidance, many acute units are still struggling to define what they do, and how they can work effectively within the 'whole systems approach' to providing mental health care.

The inpatient policy implementation guide stresses the need for the philosophy of care to be "explicitly user focused" (DH, 2002). It also quotes from an earlier Mind report in stating that the purpose of an adult acute inpatient service is "to provide a high standard of humane care in a safe and therapeutic setting for service users in the most acute and vulnerable stage of their illness. It should be for the benefit of those service users whose circumstances or acute care needs are such that they cannot at that time be treated and supported appropriately at home or in an alternative, less restrictive residential setting" (Mind, 1999).

Staff and service users from the NHS trusts participating in the *Search for Acute Solutions* project, held a series of workshops with SCMH staff to explore the role and function of acute inpatient care. The results were synthesised into the following description, taken from the unpublished SCMH report (Braithwaite, T., in Warner *et al.*, 2003) on the base-line evaluation of the project.

Box 2: The role and function of acute inpatient care

Crisis resolution: to provide rapid help and support through crisis to people with mental health problems who are severely distressed and cannot be beneficially treated/supported at home.

Safety, security and space: in a calm, dignified and homely environment – respite, asylum or sanctuary.

Assessment (including risk assessment): to provide rapid multi-disciplinary and collaborative inter-team (community and inpatient) assessment to identify service users' immediate and longer term goals, keeping the service user at the centre as the expert and focusing on their strengths as well as their needs.

Planned admissions as part of crisis prevention: for treatment and therapeutic interventions that are more beneficially provided on an inpatient basis.

Therapeutic treatment and care focused on recovery: during the inpatient stay, to start problem solving and initiate or continue a range of therapies (including therapies that are often stopped when someone is admitted), treatment and care that will set them on the road to recovery and will be continued by relevant community services. To help service users to develop affirmative attitudes to their experience.

Box 2: The role and function of acute inpatient care *(continued)*

Assertive discharge that supports community inclusion: to develop, from the time of admission, a care pathway that links the person to appropriate community resources and agencies, and supports to enable them to return home as soon as possible, ideally within two weeks. To support the maintenance of existing positive networks and links (family, friends, education, care co-ordinator, employment) to actively prevent social exclusion during the inpatient period. The range of options offered to be negotiated with and tailored to the individual person. There should be flexible levels and types of support and a focus on developing personalised relapse prevention and coping strategies and community inclusive plans that enable people to maintain and expand their skills.

Part of an integrated whole system of mental health services: For acute inpatient care to be able to become more focused, it was considered crucial that there should be a well-linked whole system of mental health care. This should provide earlier intervention to help prevent people becoming acutely distressed and would need to include well-functioning alternatives to admission in the community including crisis resolution services and home treatment for people for whom acute inpatient care is not the best option. Where admission to hospital is the most appropriate option, it should be time limited or for the shortest period required to resolve the crisis. Community and inpatient services should work together throughout admission and when planning discharge. Early discharge should be provided with sound linkages to necessary community supports (including non-mental health specific resources) to limit the likelihood of relapse and readmission and promote recovery.

This description may, perhaps, serve as a starting point for those responsible in the next 20 years for making acute care an effective and valued aspect of mental health services – an aspiration that has never been of greater importance than it is today.

4 The Mental Health Workforce

Malcolm Philip

Introduction

Mental health services are currently in the midst of huge change and expansion. As service change is being implemented, there are many workforce developments with new roles, reviews of existing roles and new types of teams. This is at a time of a significant workforce crisis, both in recruiting and retaining mental health staff now, and in creating the workforce for the future.

The last 20 years has been characterised by three phases: a period of central control of the workforce in the 1980s; opportunities for local development from 1991 to 1998 (the period of the NHS internal market and freedoms for trusts to set their own terms and conditions); and a return to strong central control since 1998. Staff across mental health and social care have seen many re-organisations, service changes, job role changes, and terms and conditions changes, and these are set to continue. Indeed the pace of change for the NHS mental health workforce has risen rapidly since the publication of the *National Service Framework (NSF) for Mental Health* (DH, 1999), the *NHS Plan* (DH, 2000a), and a raft of related policy implementation guidance. The pace of change has risen just as rapidly for social care staff in mental health, starting with *Modernising Social Services* (DH, 1998a).

The 1980s

The latter half of the 1980s in the NHS saw the introduction of 'general management' and the beginnings of 'directorate management'. 'General management' was introduced following the Griffiths report (Griffiths, 1984) which recommended moving away from committee-based management to management by senior managers and chief executives. These managers would be held individually accountable, improving the quality of management across the NHS, enabling better financial management and putting much greater emphasis on providing value for money. 'Directorate management' split organisations into large clinical groupings and, in its original form, proposed tripartite management by a nurse manager, operational manager and a lead doctor. The principle was to involve doctors more in management. For mental health staff this meant clearer accountability, a stronger management culture and, some argue, a reduction in the power and influence of professionals (Morton-Cooper & Bamford, 1997). However it developed very slowly. The role of the lead doctor was expanded in the 1990s into the Clinical Director role, but the actual managerial functions of the Clinical Director varied greatly across different hospitals.

Staff levels across England were significantly lower than today and were not growing at a fast pace. There was no expectation of service expansion, due to continued limited investment in mental health, and thus there was little need for increasing staffing. Difficulties in recruitment were appearing but health authorities responded to individual problems with little need for concerted action. In the late 1980s the first predictions appeared of a staffing crisis to come. The NHS Regional Manpower Planners Group (1988), for example, predicted serious shortages by 2001.

Staff experienced a major revision to terms and conditions. This began with nurses through the introduction of clinical grading in 1988. This replaced the previous simple grades of nursing assistant, enrolled nurse, staff nurse etc. with a new nine grade structure. This proved to be very contentious and divisive for staff and took some years to fully implement and resolve. Changes in terms and conditions for other staff groups followed.

Many organisations sought ways to increase productivity and reduce costs; common ways of doing this included lowering staff numbers on inpatient units and changing shift times and shift systems. The unions representing staff battled against many of these changes with limited success; as with the rest of British industry, this was the time of declining power for the trade unions.

The 1990s

The 1990s heralded a new system for health and social care, including mental health, with major changes to policies on the way the NHS and social care should be managed and structured. Through the 1990s the changes had an impact on all levels of staff with the introduction of the internal market, competition with the private sector, moving some services from the public to the private sector (including the staff involved), performance measurement and management, decentralised operational management, and revised payment systems (Flynn, 2002).

Health services were organised into NHS trusts in the new system and had freedom to set their own terms and conditions for staff. This had mixed results. Pay levels were maintained within strict financial limits, partly due to very tight cost control exerted on NHS trusts and partly by inertia in trusts. The unions also fought hard to uphold one of their last bastions of influence – national pay bargaining. For social services, local authorities had similar freedoms to set their own terms and conditions.

For some this meant improvements in their working lives and in their terms and conditions; for others it resulted in their department being 'contracted out' to another employer with a reduction in their benefits, pay, employment protection and union representation. In the 1990s the public sector lost its reputation of "the state as a good employer" (Flanagan, 1998).

Box 1 sets out some of the effects on terms and conditions experienced by mental health staff during this period.

Box 1: Changes in terms and conditions for mental health staff during the 1990s

Improvements for some staff

❖ Better staff numbers/teams

❖ Partnership and integrated working between NHS and social care

❖ Greater opportunities and funding for training

❖ Appraisal and supervision

❖ Skilled and supportive management

❖ Better pay, conditions and contracts

❖ Improved annual leave

❖ Improved support at work, access to counselling etc.

❖ More access to nurseries and after school care.

Worsening conditions for others

❖ Fragmented teams, overburdened with work

❖ Lack of integrated working with social care

❖ Poor management

❖ Reduced pay and conditions i.e. lessening sick pay provisions

❖ Little or no support at work

❖ A blame culture that was perceived as punitive rather than supportive

❖ Staff put on short-term contracts to match annual funding arrangements for trusts and local authorities, with potential loss of long-term employment rights

❖ Gagging clauses in contracts to stop staff speaking out

❖ Little staff involvement in organisational decision making

❖ Loss of NHS employment and provisions via 'contracting out', often matched with loss of union representation and employment protection

❖ Shortages of funding resulting in posts being frozen and greater burdens being placed on the remaining staff.

The biggest service change across mental health and social care was the long heralded move to more community based services and less inpatient based care. This included the closure of many large institutions with the consequential move of many staff into smaller homes for patients based in the community, and some staff moved into community working in outreach, day care, home based support or primary care. In local authorities the process of moving services into the private sector was greater, with many local authority-run services being contracted out. There was a need to equip staff to move into community settings and work in different team configurations with skill mixes different from those for which they were originally trained (SCMH, 1997).

These moves were often times of great anxiety for staff and patients. The quality of the change was very mixed: sometimes it was well planned with staff being well prepared and trained for their new roles; on other occasions the preparation for staff was wholly inadequate. Some staff took the opportunity to retire until it was realised that this added to the growing shortage of staff in the latter part of the 1990s.

The early part of the 1990s saw the introduction of Project 2000, moving all pre-registration nurse training into higher education. This was part of a move to make nursing a degree based profession. While this was welcomed, it did mean great change for services which had previously relied on student nurses to supplement their ward teams. At the same time the enrolled nurse training was phased out and all enrolled nurses were encouraged to undertake further training to become registered mental nurses (RMNs). Gradually two significant portions of inpatient nursing teams disappeared and services were slow to replace them.

A major ambition of the Conservative government was to reduce spending on the state (Flynn, 2002), and thus public sector budgets were tightly controlled. Services continued to run with no expectation of financial investment beyond (or even matching) the level of inflation each year. Planning for the workforce was not deemed a priority. The dire predictions made by some made back in the previous decade (e.g. Regional Manpower Planners Group, 1988), were ignored. This was in part due to the recession in the early 1990s, which lowered staff turnover and appeared to lessen staff shortages. At this time many trusts also took the decision to sell off their staff accommodation, as the lower staff turnover and buoyant levels of staffing made them believe staff accommodation was no longer required, and thus it became an asset to be sold.

In 2005, it is strange to look back ten years and read of surplus nurses in some parts of the country and of nurses being made redundant.

> "There seem to be new reports of nurses facing redundancy almost weekly, newly qualified staff nurses looking at short and sometimes very short-term contracts, or the prospect of unemployment" (Mangan, 1994).

Numbers required to enter pre-registration training were also reduced across many professions, as planning was based on the current situation without looking ahead. This was only reversed in the late 1990s when the staffing crisis for health and social care had already begun. By that time the cost of living in some parts of the country was becoming prohibitive for public sector workers, which added to the recruitment difficulties for organisations in those areas.

The predictions of shortages of staff, ignored through the 1990s, turned out to be accurate. By the end of the decade there were serious staffing shortages which had an impact on both service users and permanent staff. In 2000, the Sainsbury Centre for Mental Health stated that there were vacancy levels of 14% for consultant psychiatrists, 85% of trusts reporting difficulties in filling nursing posts, shortfalls of clinical psychologists, and 10% vacancy levels for occupational therapists across the NHS. Social work vacancy levels were not quantifiable although authorities reported shortages (SCMH, 2000).

Services suffered from understaffing and high turnover which affected quality of care for users and sent services into a vicious circle. Staff did not have enough time, or colleagues, to improve their practice. They were trying to cope with too much work which in turn could lead to them leaving. In response to staff shortages, some services made heavy use of agency staff and locums. This was expensive, destabilising to mental health teams, and made it much more difficult to ensure that a high quality and safe service was provided (SCMH, 2000).

No planning for the mental health workforce had been undertaken in the decade. As there was no expectation of any expansion of services, staffing decisions and future planning decisions were made purely by considering the situation at the time, with no analysis of future school leavers, career options, labour markets, economic factors or demand for the workforce. This was compounded by serious weaknesses, both locally and nationally, in the data on the mental health workforce. By 1999 there was still no comprehensive data on the mental health workforce in England. In 1999, the House of Commons Select Committee on Health regretted this situation and recommended radical change to workforce planning across the NHS. The NHS responded in 2000 by publishing *A Health Service of all the Talents* (DH, 2000b).

In response to the loss of staff, students, and the intermediate enrolled nurse grade some organisations began to experiment with new roles e.g. replacing the enrolled nurse grade with a new trained support role, the healthcare assistant. Similar social work support roles emerged. A few organisations began to extend the role of nurses, explore the contribution of psychologists in roles outside the clinical psychologist, and create other new specialist roles for staff, e.g. behaviour therapists. However the bulk of mental health services struggled to get beyond focusing on the current recruitment and retention crisis, and did not consider changing the nature of their workforce.

Whilst Project 2000 for nursing was generally viewed as successful, it was not without its problems. In the latter part of the 1990s some organisations began to call for a set of competencies for mental health staff and the modernisation of training to reflect the changes happening in the way services were delivered, (e.g. SCMH 1997). As community based services increased, so different approaches for different client groups developed, formalised by legislative changes and policy developments. Staff needed to adhere to these new policies, while taking into account the new focus on choice and on the perspectives of users and carers. This required new skill sets for staff which higher education was often not well equipped to provide, and to which it is still finding difficulty adjusting today.

A key issue to address in the move to a greater emphasis on service provision in the community was the notion of multidisciplinary working in community based teams, as health and social care came together to provide seamless care. Multidisciplinary teamworking denoted that each team member had special skills to contribute to the care of patients and that these contributions were made in conjunction with others, leading to common goals in delivering the service. Again the results were very mixed, ranging from fully integrated community teams to entirely separated groups of professionals in the same service, where no integration or common understanding had been achieved (Rogers & Pilgrim, 2001).

With the major changes to the NHS in the 1980s and 1990s there was a decentralisation of management and delegation of responsibilities to local level. As Farnham and Horton (1996) state, the NHS moved away from being a 'model employer' to one concerned with efficiency and effective performance. There was an expectation that local HR directors and teams would lead a positive agenda for the workforce. Some commentators and surveys did discern some development of the personnel function into a more strategic role and some evidence of more progressive HR practices being employed (Barnett *et al.*, 1996).

However a common theme of many commentators, including Bach (1998), was that some of the expectations of change had not been realised, as managers were constrained in their autonomy to act at local level. Constraints identified included national policy and central government intervention; the embedded mechanisms for determining terms and conditions nationally; and the determination of expenditure by government coupled with the difficulties in funding at the local level.

The development of a strategic HR agenda locally had not developed as much as expected given the freedoms created for managers, and in 1997 there was a central drive with a first national HR strategy published in 1998 (DH, 1998c). This had three strategic aims: ensuring a quality workforce; improving the quality of working life for staff; and boosting the management (principally HR) capacity and capability required to deliver this agenda.

A whole range of national initiatives were begun intended to improve recruitment, retention, morale and the effectiveness of staff.

The Department of Health later followed this with a new HR strategy, *HR in the NHS Plan* (DH, 2002a). It draws together all the existing initiatives into one overall new strategy with the goal of "more staff, working differently". The principal areas covered in the strategy were: being a best practice employer; modernising pay; changing professional regulatory frameworks; improving training and development; improving staff morale; and improving the HR function.

A change of pace for the end of the century

The change of government in 1997 signalled a new direction for health and social care. Initially this did not include major financial investment, as the new Government committed itself to maintaining the previous Government's tight financial control. However as policy documents were published they showed a change of direction and a commitment to a system that was convenient, allowed patient choice, responded quickly and efficiently, and provided comprehensive, high quality services.

The NHS moved away from the internal market, emphasised quality and health improvement, introduced key action plans across areas of health (*National Service Frameworks*), and initiated stronger partnerships between agencies involved in health and social care. Structural change was widespread, including merging NHS trusts to form larger units, the development of primary care trusts (PCTs), the introduction of strategic health authorities (SHAs), changes to regional health authorities, and the creation of new bodies to take forward new plans for services nationally.

Modernising Mental Health Services, published in 1998, set out the Government's vision for future mental health services and emphasised three key aims of safe, sound and supportive services (DH, 1998b). *The National Service Framework for Mental Health* (DH, 1999) and the *NHS Plan* (DH, 2000a) set out the Government's programme of reform and investment to provide comprehensive adult mental health services across the country. Further *National Service Frameworks* have followed for older people (DH, 2001b) and children's services (DH, 2004a) which include mental health and social care provision. The services were to be planned around and sensitive to the needs of the service users and carers. *The Mental Health Policy Implementation Guide* was published in 2001 to guide trusts in the adult services they needed to set up, the format of those services and some information about potential staffing (DH, 2001a). The guide envisaged full scale implementation of the *NSF* and *NHS Plan* between 2002 and 2004.

In April 2002 the Government announced further steps on investment and reform. There would be major investment with an overall target of health spending to reach 9.4% of GDP

(Gross Domestic Product) by 2008, on a par with European levels of spending. Investment was planned to grow by 7.5% per annum up to 2008, with mental health services expecting their portion of this to allow the full implementation of the *NSF* (DH, 2002b).

Social services were also to be transformed with the Department of Health modernisation programme, *Modernising Social Services* (1998a). The modernisation agenda sought to promote independence, improve consistency, and provide convenient, user focused services. It aimed also to improve protection; boost standards in the workforce; support partnership working between health and social services; and improve delivery. As with the NHS, though to a lesser extent, with this agenda came extra funding.

Critical to achieving this modernised comprehensive mental health and social care service was increased staffing. As each element of modernisation is introduced through service change or proposed legislation, each seems to require yet more staff. Estimates vary from 10,000 to over 30,000 new staff to fully implement the modernisation across mental health and social care. The Department of Health recognised this and promised greater investment in all the key professions in mental health. However it should be remembered that this required huge expansion came at a time when the Department of Health was implementing policy initiatives across all health and social care sectors, necessitating staffing expansion in each one. This began when the NHS and social care services already faced a serious staffing crisis and an ageing workforce.

Mental health services suddenly needed to shift from staffing to maintain the existing mental health service provision, to finding ways to staff a rapidly expanding service. As the planning to maintain the existing workforce was woeful, meeting the Department of Health demand for an expanded service looked very ambitious. Indeed many, including SCMH, argued that the staffing expansion required was unachievable, based on the current models of delivering care. New ways of working needed to be explored urgently and new ways of staffing services found.

The need to address the staffing issues was recognised nationally and a national underpinning programme on workforce planning, education and training for adult mental health was established: the Workforce Action Team (WAT). The aim of the WAT programme was "to enable mental health services to ensure that their workforce is sufficient and skilled, well led and supported to deliver high quality mental health care, including secure mental health care" (Workforce Action Team, 2001). The WAT sought to develop a national picture of the staff needed to deliver the *NSF* and *NHS Plan*; how they might be recruited and retained; what education and training should be available; what skills or competencies they would need; and what the skill mix of the future workforce should be.

The final WAT report was published in 2001 (Workforce Action Team, 2001) and made recommendations about:

❖ The recruitment and retention of staff

- ❖ National occupational standards for all staff working in mental health services

- ❖ A single agreed set of the knowledge, skills and attitudes required by the mental health practitioner workforce

- ❖ Employing skill mix solutions to provide an adequate workforce

- ❖ Recruiting more trained support staff into the mental health workforce

- ❖ Developing a range of models assessing the potential numbers and mix of staff required to deliver the *NSF* and the *NHS Plan* at a national level

- ❖ Addressing primary mental health care workforce issues

- ❖ Mapping all current education and training provision

- ❖ A programme of engagement with the professional and regulatory bodies, to discuss the outcome of the mapping exercise in relation to pre-qualification training and continuing professional development

- ❖ Tackling the stigma which is attached to working in mental health services.

This work is currently being taken forward by the Workforce Implementation Team, the Mental Health Care Group Workforce Team, and the National Institute for Mental Health England (NIMHE) and its regional development centres. Associated work has been led by the NHS Changing Workforce Programme, the Modernisation Agency and the Topss England new roles project. Projects are underway in all the areas identified above as services seek ways of staffing the expansion.

The new roles conceived during the last decade in response to staffing difficulties have influenced the development of some of the new roles being explored now; for example there are similarities between the NVQ qualified Senior Healthcare Assistant of the 1990s and the new Support, Time and Recovery worker (who provides non-clinical support to service users and helps them towards recovery). Other roles being piloted are very new, such as Gateway workers (designed to help GPs manage and treat common mental health problems in all age groups), and Community Development workers (who help to improve the experience of people from Black and minority ethnic communities using mental health services). The emphasis and national support given to explore new ways of working is very welcome, as are the large and diverse projects being led by the various agencies, particularly NIMHE both nationally and through the regional development centres. Existing roles are also being reviewed and pilots developed to look at new ways of working for existing staff and teams, for example on the role of the consultant psychiatrist.

Training and education are being reviewed and updated to provide future staff with the skills to run the modernised services. *The Capable Practitioner Framework* (SCMH, 2001), *The Ten Essential Shared Capabilities* (NIMHE 2004), the national occupational standards for health and social care (Skills for Health, 2003), the *NHS Knowledge and Skills*

Framework (DH, 2004b), the NHS job evaluation scheme for the new NHS pay scheme (DH, 2004c), and *Modernising the Social Care Workforce* (Topss England, 2000) are all connected to devising future staff roles, capabilities and skills.

However, the training and education agenda described above also shows that there is almost too much being developed and too many overlapping initiatives. This is not unique to training and education but is common across mental health. In the 1990s there were few national initiatives or projects, with a reliance on trusts and local authorities to develop things for themselves; now there are too many organisations working on too many similar projects, with no coherent overall framework for change. To provide one example, the new NHS pay system takes no account of pay structures in social care, even though integration of social care and NHS mental health services are a top priority with many social care staff now under the management of the NHS. There has been a bewildering array of working groups, taskforces, action teams and guidance documents on developing workforce issues (Genkeer *et al.*, 2003).

The recruitment and retention crisis has not improved since the 1990s and in many parts of the country the crisis has deepened. All the problems identified in the 1990s are still prevalent today. In its review of the *NSF* after five years, the Department of Health points out that staffing figures have improved, for example from 1999-2003 consultant psychiatrist numbers increased by 25%, nurses 13% and clinical psychologists 42%, but admits that vacancies remain a serious problem (DH, 2004d).

Both recruitment and retention are significant problems for many trusts and local authorities. In the NHS, an ageing workforce, violence against staff, stress, overburdening workloads and role clarity are just some of the challenges. The high cost of living in some areas exacerbates the problems. Inpatient services suffer particularly from staff shortages, high turnover, overuse of bank and agency staff and low morale. This is the picture Genkeer *et al.* (2003) describe in London and it is replicated for many mental health services across the country.

Similar problems are reported in social work. According to Huxley *et al.* (2003), 43% of mental health social workers feel undervalued at work. Volume of work, poor administrative support, poor management, physically unacceptable accommodation, and shared offices make their jobs difficult. These issues contribute to recruitment and retention problems: 72% of social work managers report problems recruiting approved social workers; and only 17% of social workers feel positively about the place of social work in modern mental health services.

These recruitment and retention problems are reflected in the Commission for Health Improvement report on mental health trusts (CHI, 2003). The local experience varied with some trusts having high morale, good communication and strong management and clinical relationships; whereas other trusts had poor staffing levels, low morale, stress, high workloads and poor communication between staff and management. These same issues are highlighted across the public sector by the Audit Commission (2002).

Along with all the factors identified relating to recruitment and retention problems, pay is becoming critical. Pay across mental health professions has not kept pace with other public sector roles and lags well behind comparative private sector pay rates. Full-time social workers' pay is at the bottom end of the range for professional occupations (Topss England, 2003), with only librarians and the clergy earning less. Social workers' pay is broadly similar to nurses' pay. Pay levels have seriously drifted in the last ten years and it is essential this is reversed so that mental health professions do not become 'low pay professions'.

What of the future?

The work underway through the Workforce Implementation Team, NIMHE and the associated work through other national bodies is vital to recruit and retain staff, explore new ways of working for existing professionals and develop and validate new roles and training and education. This work is explained in the *National Mental Health Workforce Strategy* (DH, 2004e). Many trusts are involved in aspects of the work, although more NHS trusts need to become involved and implement a whole range of changes not just single projects focused on individual jobs. All the work is aimed at modernising and expanding the workforce. Yet it remains questionable whether all of the efforts thus far described are sufficient to deal with the scale of the challenge.

Given the combination of serious staff shortages and very large expansion that is needed to create comprehensive mental health services across England, it is probably not possible to find all the staff that are required. The pressure to find new staff, moreover, is compounded by the need to create new staff roles across health and social care to achieve the Government's broad goals for them.

Trusts and local authorities are still very poor at planning and developing their future workforce, which is part of the reason for the current shortages. There seems to be very slow movement towards proper planning of the workforce, funding the creation of that workforce and producing challenging and satisfying jobs for staff.

It is possible that the forecast workforce expansion required will turn out to be overestimated. If health and social care funding continues to go disproportionately to other parts of the service and not reach mental health providers, then their planned expansion will be curtailed and thus workforce requirements curtailed.

SCMH (2003) outlined five possible approaches to solving the staffing gap for the future – see Figure 1.

Figure 1: Addressing the gaps

Cultural shift

1. Deciding to take no action

2. Making the best use of current resources

3. How to enhance current resources

4. Innovative solutions

5. An integrated economy approach

Integration with community

Deciding to take no action is not a realistic option, although some trusts could be described as being in this position. In many places, systems have not been in place to record and analyse workforce information, changes of staff and posts have been inadequately monitored, and so staffing shortages have not been understood. Deciding to take no action now will add to the shortages and undermine mental health service modernisation.

Considering how to make the best use of resources and how to enhance current resources are the two approaches on which most of the nationally led effort is being concentrated. Current efforts include investigating better ways of using existing staff, creating new roles and revising existing ones supported by new and updated training and education. Areas needing more priority are the creation of a truly diverse workforce, bringing users and carers into mental health employment, and making better use of different labour markets e.g. refugees.

It is essential that, in addition to all of this activity, more innovative solutions are considered and tested out. If supply cannot match staffing demand, can the demand be changed? This necessitates more radical rethinks of service delivery, including thinking beyond current structures and limitations. More options need to be tried with greater involvement of the voluntary sector, user-led services and the private sector. This could include reviews of existing parts of the service or complete reassessments of how services are delivered.

The last of the approaches, that of the integrated economy, is perhaps the most difficult. Historically the statutory sector has planned services focusing mainly on statutory sector provision. An integrated economy approach would take an inclusive perspective on the whole mental health economy, with all agencies deciding how to make the best use of their resources together. *The Mental Health Policy Implementation Guide* (DH, 2001a) argued for a whole systems approach. This means going beyond ensuring the inclusion of the full range of agencies in service planning. It means looking at the overall systems and structures for delivering mental health and social care, and the needs of the community they serve, including groups or individuals with unmet need, and planning the workforce from there.

The challenge is whether mental health and social care services organisations, PCTs, SHAs, local authorities, the Department of Health and associated bodies can succeed with an often stated goal: "having the right staff with the right skills in the right place at the right time".

Table 1: Mental Health Workforce in England, 1982-2003				
STAFF TYPE	**1982**	**1991**	**1999**	**2003**
Consultant psychiatrists	1,360	1,675.4	2,524	3,155
Mental health nurses	19,110	27,010	34,974	39,383
Enrolled nurses	12,110	7,990	*	*
Unqualified	16,590	18,010	NPA	NPA
Clinical psychologists	1,180	2,330	3,763	5,331
Support	NPA	NPA	550	1,070
Occupational therapists**	3,180	5,630	10,792	13,053
Support	NPA	NPA	1,934	2,013
Social workers	NPA	NPA	7,500	9,700
Psychotherapists	NPA	NPA	365	631
Support	NPA	NPA	16	63

Notes

* Enrolled nurses grade phased out

** Occupational therapy numbers are generic, not mental health-specific

NPA – No published figures available

All figures in whole time equivalents (WTEs). The table provides an outline picture only as figures previously collected did not identify staff in mental health separately.

For sources of these figures, see References.

5 The Mental Health Economy

Michael Parsonage

Introduction

The last 20 years have seen extensive changes in the policy and organisational framework that governs the provision of mental health care. Some of these changes reflect NHS-wide processes of reform, while others have been specific to mental health. The pace and scale of change have, if anything, been greater in the second half of the period than in the first. Also, the level of public spending on mental health care has risen substantially over the period and again the increases have been bigger in the later years than in the earlier ones.

These changes have undoubtedly resulted in more and better services for people with mental health problems, yet serious concerns persist. Few would deny, for example, that standards of care still often fall well short of those in other parts of the NHS. The physical environment in which much psychiatric inpatient care is provided would be regarded as unacceptable in general acute hospitals, while the lengthy waiting times for treatment that are now increasingly a thing of the past for elective services remain commonplace in mental health.

The easy explanation of such concerns is to say that, despite the increased availability of resources, mental heath care remains seriously under-funded. While not questioning that more expenditure would be welcome, this chapter argues that analysis of the mental health economy should also pay close heed to the ways in which available resources are used. Mental health services may or may not be under-funded but they are almost certainly under-managed. Debate on how best to improve the overall effectiveness of care needs to strike a new balance between the sufficiency of resources on the one hand and the efficiency of their use on the other.

One reason why mental health care is under-managed has been the sheer scale of policy and organisational change confronting those responsible for running services in recent years. Over the last two decades the system has on the whole been policy-led rather than management-led. Looking to the future, the best way of making sustained improvements in services may well be to reverse this order of priorities.

Recent developments in the mental health economy

Reliable and consistent data on the evolution of total NHS and social service spending on mental health care is not readily available because of changes in accounting definitions and gaps in coverage. For example, it is commonly reckoned that of all people coming into contact with the NHS because of mental health problems, about 90% are dealt with in primary care, without subsequent referral to specialist services (Goldberg & Huxley, 1992). Despite this, no information is routinely available on the costs of mental health care provided by GPs or other primary care staff. Looking ahead, such problems should be solved by the Department of Health's National Programme Budget project, which – at least for future years – will provide a comprehensive analysis of NHS expenditure by medical condition (DH, 2004a).

For historical analysis, the best that can be done is to focus on spending trends in the secondary or specialist mental health services funded by the NHS and in the services for people with mental health problems paid for by local authority social service departments.

Information published by the Department of Health indicates that in 1984/85 combined expenditure on these services in England amounted to £1,160 million, while in 2003/04 the corresponding total was £5,687 million (DHSS, 1986; DH, 2004a, 2004b). (The figure for 1984/85 includes a small amount of spending on residential care funded by social security payments that were transferred to local authorities in 1993.) These totals are in current or 'out-turn' prices and so do not allow for inflation. Using the NHS pay and prices index as an appropriate deflator, it is calculated that the total spending increase in inflation-adjusted or volume terms was 86.9% over the period, corresponding to an average growth rate of 3.3% a year.

Further analysis indicates that, again allowing for NHS pay and price inflation, aggregate spending on mental health services increased by 22.4% in the years between 1984/85 and 1994/95 but by 52.7% in the years between 1994/95 and 2003/04. These increases translate into average growth rates of 2.0% and 4.8% a year respectively. In other words, annual expenditure on mental health care grew more than twice as fast in the second half of the period as in the first.

It is also worth noting that, over the period as a whole, expenditure on mental health care grew slightly more rapidly than spending on other services provided by the NHS and local authorities and so increased its share of the overall budget for health and social care. Thus the proportion of total spending on NHS hospital and community health services devoted to mental health rose from 11.3% to 12.6% between 1984/85 and 2003/04, while in the case of local authority spending on social services the share of mental health increased from 3.2% to 5.4%.

The way this money was spent changed in two important ways. First, the balance of expenditure between the NHS and social services shifted, with the share of the latter increasing from 6% of the total in 1984/85 to 15% in 2003/04. Second, there was a decline in the relative importance of hospital inpatient services, from 78% of overall spending in 1984/85 to 49% in 2003/04. Both these changes reflect the continuing shift towards community-based care that has been a broad objective of policy throughout the period.

Developments in the organisational and management framework for mental health care are less easily summarised, as the period under review has been one of almost continuous change. This particularly reflects the frequency of structural reorganisations in the NHS (and, to a lesser extent, local government) and other programmes of management reform.

An abbreviated list of key changes in organisation and management is as follows:

❖ The introduction of an internal market in the NHS following the 1989 White Paper *Working for Patients* (DH, 1989), the crucial enduring feature of which has been an organisational split between those responsible for commissioning and purchasing health services and those responsible for providing them.

❖ Continuing evolution of commissioning structures, reflecting among other things the difficulty of striking the right balance between the advantages of small scale (e.g. closeness to service users) and those of large scale (e.g. purchasing clout).

❖ Similar structural changes on the provider side, including the creation of self-governing NHS trusts and latterly the emergence of increasingly large, multi-site specialist mental health trusts, as a result of mergers and other reorganisations.

❖ More joint working between NHS and local authority agencies, particularly following the Health Act 1999, which allowed the introduction of pooled budgets, joint commissioning and integrated provision of services.

❖ The growth of a mixed economy of care, which in the case of mental health has been reflected in an increasingly large proportion of publicly funded services being supplied on contract by independent and voluntary sector providers.

❖ A succession of NHS-wide initiatives on performance management and clinical governance, all aimed at raising standards and improving accountability but with varying degrees of emphasis on central control as against local autonomy.

Other changes still to come or at an early stage of implementation include practice-based commissioning, new arrangements for patient choice, the introduction of Foundation Trusts and payment by results. All of these are likely to have important but as yet unresolved implications for mental health.

Continuing problems

Investment and modernisation have undoubtedly raised the profile of mental health issues and brought about substantial improvements in the quantity and quality of care. Yet both official and unofficial reports continue to paint a picture of mixed performance and enduring concerns. The following extracts from a report on mental health trusts published in December 2003 by the Commission for Health Improvement (CHI), now the Healthcare Commission, are representative:

> "The historical legacy of the neglect of mental health services is still regrettably evident in the findings of CHI's investigations...Trusts and services are at very different stages of development...A number of trusts are performing well, but a larger number face significant challenges...Despite a broad consensus about mental health policy, wide engagement with the agenda and evidence of innovation and change, there is considerable dissatisfaction in the mental health sector that the priority accorded to mental health is not always reflected in practice...Factors such as the isolation of services, institutional environments, low staffing levels and high use of bank and agency staff, closed cultures and poor clinical leadership and supervision have caused the neglect of patients...CHI's reviews show that mental health services, despite the progress evident over the period of our reviews, still lag some way behind the acute sector..." (CHI, 2003a).

Drawing on such evidence, continuing areas of concern in the mental health economy can be grouped together under three main headings.

Variations

The CHI report is primarily a review of clinical governance and it describes in some detail wide differences between mental health trusts in the development and effectiveness of their management systems. This is, however, only one aspect of variability in the mental health economy. Others include substantial geographical differences in levels of spending on mental health care and in the availability of services (Glover & Barnes, 2003) and also variations between providers in the unit costs of service provision over and above those attributable to differences in input prices (DH, 2004c).

Geographical variations in provision may be illustrated by reference to a recent report on financing mental health services in London (Aziz *et al.*, 2003). This found that among London's 32 boroughs per capita spending on NHS mental health services in 2001/02 ranged from £41 to £160, while spending per head on mental health services by local authorities varied between £16 and £82. Statistical analysis showed that differences in need could account for some of this variation, but a good deal remained unexplained.

Thus a comparison of actual spending on NHS services with the level predicted on the basis of need found that the highest spending borough spent 29% per head more than expected, while the lowest spending borough spent 59% less than expected (Aziz *et al.*, 2003). These differences in resource availability are larger than those found in the funding of general acute services.

Shortfalls in provision

Shortfalls in service provision can be described and assessed in various ways. Three aspects are noted here.

First, epidemiological surveys consistently find evidence of high levels of unmet need for mental health treatment in the general population. For example, a recent study of general practice attenders found that while the overall prevalence of mental health problems in the sample was 27.3%, more than half of this group (59.6%) had unmet needs and a further 6.2% had partially met needs (Boardman *et al.*, 2004). The prevalence of unmet need was highest among those with anxiety disorders.

Second, there is evidence that standards of care in mental health often fall below those in other parts of the NHS. This is hard to justify, given the equity principle on which the NHS is based. As an example, sustained efforts have been made in recent years to reduce waiting lists in the acute hospital sector, including the use of increasingly demanding targets. No such targets have ever been set for mental health services and in many cases systematic information on waiting lists and waiting times is not even collected. Such evidence as is available often suggests extremely lengthy waits, especially for psychological therapies where two-year waits are "not uncommon" (Forrest, 2004).

Third, the resources being made available for mental health care are not growing rapidly enough to deliver the Government's declared policy objectives. According to Department of Health estimates published in the Wanless Review of long-term health spending, implementation of the *National Service Framework for Mental Health* (DH, 1999) requires annual real terms increases in expenditure on mental health services of 8.8% a year between 2002/03 and 2010/11 (Wanless, 2001; 2002). The available evidence does not suggest that spending is currently growing at the required rate, implying a widening gap between plan and performance in the delivery of better care (SCMH, 2003a).

Inefficiencies

Economic analysis draws a distinction between two aspects of efficiency: technical efficiency (producing a given level of output at minimum cost) and allocative efficiency (producing an economically appropriate mix or combination of outputs). In everyday language the distinction is between doing things right and doing the right things. Both aspects are relevant in the present context.

Hard evidence on the scale of technical inefficiency in the provision of mental health care is in short supply, partly reflecting the lack of good information on costs and outputs. But anecdotal evidence suggests that it is substantial. The wide and unexplained variations in unit costs between mental health providers point in the same direction, as do the general findings of audit reports and similar reviews.

Firmer conclusions can perhaps be drawn from the evidence on inappropriate referrals and placements, as this almost certainly indicates a waste or misuse of resources. Research studies have found that up to 28% of referrals from primary care to specialist mental health services are inappropriate (cited in Social Exclusion Unit, 2004). Up to a third of admissions to acute inpatient psychiatric care are inappropriate and, when delayed discharges as well as inappropriate admissions are taken into account, up to 58% of hospital bed use is inappropriate (Glasby & Lester, 2003a). It is also estimated that between 37% and 75% of patients in high security hospitals may not need the services provided there, and in one medium secure unit only 45% of patients were appropriately placed (Glasby & Lester, 2003b). Some of these findings may need modification in the light of recent developments in service provision, but there is little doubt that the problem of inappropriate placements remains substantial.

Turning to allocative efficiency, two commonly noted areas of concern are: first, that the balance of resources available for mental health care is disproportionately skewed towards those with serious mental health problems at the expense of the much larger numbers with common disorders such as anxiety and depression; and second, that the mental health system is very much a sickness system, with insufficient attention given on the one hand to prevention and health promotion and on the other to recovery, rehabilitation and employment.

To elaborate briefly, the main focus of mental health policy is on the care of people with severe and enduring illness and in consequence the great bulk of resources are directed at specialist treatment. At any one time the number of people in touch with these services is around 630,000 (NIMHE, 2004). However, epidemiological surveys show prevalence rates of 15-25% for all mental disorders in the adult population, or up to 10 million people in England (ONS, 2002). Spending is thus concentrated heavily on a sub-group which includes only around 1 in 12 of all those with mental health needs. There is little clear evidence that this makes sense in either human or economic terms.

Similar concerns apply to the balance of expenditure between the treatment and care of mental illness on the one hand and other forms of intervention such as prevention, health promotion and rehabilitation on the other. The *National Service Framework for Mental Health* (DH, 1999) includes a standard for promotion, but the resources available for its implementation have so far been scarce: according to recent evidence just 0.1% of mental health service spending is devoted to mental health promotion (SCMH, 2003a). More is being done in the area of rehabilitation and re-employment, but the scale of the problem is huge. There are now nearly one million people claiming Incapacity Benefit because of mental health problems, almost twice as many as ten years ago, and the employment rate among those with long-term mental health problems is the lowest for any of the main groups of disabled people (Social Exclusion Unit, 2004). It has been estimated that the total cost of lost output resulting from the impact of mental illness on people's capacity to work amounted to £23.1 billion in 2002/03 (SCMH, 2003b). This is about three times as much as the total amount spent on mental health care by the NHS and local authorities.

Weaknesses in planning, organisation and management

In analysing these shortcomings, most observers give considerable weight to a historical legacy of neglect and under-funding, typified by the statement in the Wanless Review that "For far too long, mental health has been stigmatised and starved of resources and national attention" (Wanless, 2001). Financial constraints cannot, however, easily explain all of the problems noted above, particularly those relating to variability in performance and inefficiencies in the use and allocation of available resources. Other considerations also come into play, and prominent among these are important unresolved weaknesses in the planning, organisation and management of mental health services.

Evidence for such weaknesses is documented in the reports of inspectorates such as the Audit Commission and the Commission for Health Improvement (CHI). These reveal a range of shortcomings in the management capacity of mental health trusts and a level of organisational performance that generally lags behind that in most other parts of the NHS.

Star ratings

Star ratings have been published for mental health trusts in 2003 and 2004, with performance being assessed against a range of targets and indicators (CHI, 2003b; Healthcare Commission, 2004). Many of these measures relate to organisation and management. While subject to various limitations, the ratings system does offer some comparisons with trusts in the acute sector. Such comparisons confirm the relatively poor performance of mental health trusts. For example, the figures for 2004 show that twice as many mental health trusts obtained one or zero stars as obtained three stars (30 compared with 15), whereas among acute trusts these proportions were reversed (39 compared with 76). Along with a doubling in the number of mental health trusts awarded zero stars in 2004 compared with the previous year, such findings have led the Healthcare Commission to observe that the performance of mental health trusts remains "a cause for concern".

CHI reviews of clinical governance

The CHI report on mental health trusts quoted earlier in this chapter includes summary information on 32 completed clinical governance reviews (CHI, 2003a). Clinical governance is defined as "the framework through which NHS organisations and their staff are accountable for the quality of patient care". Seven components are assessed on a scale from 1 ("little or no progress...") to 4 ("excellence..."). The performance of the 32 mental health trusts is shown in Table 1.

Table 1: Performance of mental health trusts	Number of trusts at each level of performance			
	1	**2**	**3**	**4**
Patient and public involvement	7	22	3	0
Risk management	9	23	0	0
Clinical audit	12	18	2	0
Staffing and staff management	10	20	2	0
Education and training	3	26	3	0
Clinical effectiveness	13	17	1	1
Use of information	18	13	1	0

These ratings indicate not only a low average level of performance but also consistently weak performance across all seven components of clinical governance assessed in the reviews. In every case at least 90% of mental health trusts are in the lower half of the scale.

Audit Commission review

The Audit Commission published a report in 2003 on *Achieving the NHS Plan* (Audit Commission, 2003). Auditors assessed the progress of every trust in England towards meeting the key targets set out in the NHS Plan. The report also identified constraints on performance and assessed the strengths and weaknesses of management. Among its key conclusions was that mental health trusts showed the most weaknesses in both performance and management capacity across the board. Auditors identified management capacity issues of 'high risk' concern in as many as two-thirds of all mental health trusts. Particular shortcomings were identified in financial management.

Similar weaknesses have also been highlighted in the performance of those bodies responsible for commissioning mental health services. For example, a recent review in London by the King's Fund reported that "Weak commissioning of mental health services by primary care trusts emerged as a key factor in the slow pace of modernisation of London's mental health services" (Levenson *et al.*, 2003). Similar findings have been noted in reports with national coverage (for example, SCMH, 2003a).

The changing policy and organisational framework

These management problems among both commissioners and providers are open to a range of explanations, but their widespread nature suggests that attention should focus on factors applying across the mental health sector rather than on those of more local concern. One such candidate is the extent of change in the national policy and organisational framework for mental health care. As emphasised throughout this chapter, such change has been extensive and continuous.

Two adverse consequences can be identified. First, the persistent demands of implementing policy and organisational change have deflected management attention from the routine day-to-day task of running services as efficiently as possible. Organisational change is particularly distracting, as managers and other staff need time to settle into new posts and to establish new roles and relationships. These problems are compounded if reorganisation is preceded by a period of uncertainty about possible job losses or other adverse effects on working conditions. All of these problems have been noted in the case of mental health.

Second, some of the changes in policy and organisation have been counter-productive in their effects on the efficiency of service provision, whether because of unintended consequences or as a result of faulty design. An example of this is the emergent organisational structure of the mental health economy. There is an increasing imbalance between commissioners and providers. Commissioners have tended to get smaller over time while providers have got larger, to the point where there are currently around 300 PCTs responsible for commissioning services from only about 80 mental health provider trusts. The balance of market power is now heavily tilted towards providers, and the capacity of commissioners to promote change and overcome any provider resistance is greatly limited by a lack of contestability for services, the limited purchasing power of individual PCTs and difficulties in getting access to information held by providers.

In addition to distorting the market, the large size of mental health trusts has other adverse effects. These include remoteness from local populations (some providers now have catchment areas covering more than a million people) and costs resulting from the merging of previously separate institutions (for example, incompatible IT systems). The emergence of very large trusts has resulted from organisational changes such as the introduction of Care Trusts that combine health and social services in a single body. Such changes have generally been encouraged, and in some cases actively promoted, by central government, but the transitional and other costs of reorganisation have undoubtedly been substantial and little if any evidence has been produced to justify the new structures. The welcome emphasis now given to an evidence-based approach to mental health policy and service development does not appear to be replicated in the area of organisation and structure.

Conclusion

Mental health has long been described as a Cinderella service. Those wishing to argue that this label is no longer appropriate can point to a number of important changes in recent years. These include: the priority status attached to mental health in statements of government policy on health and social care; the early introduction of a *National Service Framework for Mental Health* (DH, 1999); and substantial increases in resources, on average since 1985 running ahead of those in the rest of the NHS and social services.

Yet it is clear that much remains to be done. Progress in the development of new and improved services has been patchy around the country. There remain gaps in provision and shortfalls in the quality of care compared with other parts of the NHS. There also remain serious concerns about the use and allocation of resources, particularly relating to the appropriate balance of spending between different groups of people with mental health needs and between different forms of service provision.

The traditional response to such concerns is to call for further increases in funding. On the Government's own figures, delivery of the policy objectives set out in the *National Service Framework* will indeed require substantial extra resources. Such increases are a necessary but not sufficient condition for the sustained improvement of mental health care. Other changes are also needed, among both commissioners and providers, in planning, organisation and management. Until the systems and processes of management in mental health match those in the rest of the NHS, the Cinderella label will be hard to shake off.

6 From Little Acorns
– The mental health service user movement

Peter Campbell

Introduction

In the summer of 1985, service user activists from the United Kingdom met activists from other countries at the Mind/World Federation of Mental Health Congress in Brighton, a coming together that underlined the potential for collective campaigning in this country. That autumn's Annual Mind Conference in Kensington Town Hall was the first national mental health event at which service users made a significant contribution to the programme.

The following year, in January 1986, Survivors Speak Out, the first national network for service users involved in action, was established. At this time, Nottingham Patients' Council Support Group was beginning its work, pioneering collective and individual advocacy. By the end of 1987, National Voices, a service user network within the National Schizophrenia Fellowship (now Rethink) and Mindlink, a similar network within Mind, were up and running and Survivors Speak Out had organised the first national conference of service user activists over a weekend at Edale Youth Hostel. It could well be said that something exciting was beginning to get underway (Wallcraft *et al.*, 2003).

It is tempting to identify the mid-1980s as the time when service user action really started. While there is a great deal of truth in such a view, it does not do justice to action that had taken place before this point. Protest against the mental health system – and protest has usually been a powerful force behind service user action – has occurred ever since the creation of the asylums nearly two hundred years ago. But for a long time protest was, more often than not, emerging from individuals rather than organised groups.

In the 1970s an important group did form. The Mental Patients Union, with branches in various parts of the country, can justifiably be called the originator of organised service user action (Crossley, 1999). When it broke up it was succeeded by a number of smaller groups: Community Organisation for Psychiatric Emergencies (COPE), Protection of the Rights of Mental Patients in Therapy (PROMPT) and Campaign Against Psychiatric Oppression (CAPO). These groups provided a link between action in the 1970s and developments in the 1980s. CAPO, for example, although quite a small group, was influential in the early 1980s and continued its work into the 1990s. A number of activists who pioneered new groups in the mid-1980s were introduced to action by the above groups and by the British Network for Alternatives to Psychiatry (BNAP), an organisation of mental health professionals and service users that had links with the 'anti-psychiatry' movement. If the real flowering of service user action took place in the late 1980s and 1990s, it was through the work of these often-neglected groups that the first seeds were sown.

Nevertheless, it is quite clear that there have been huge changes in the role of people with a mental illness diagnosis over the last 20 years – at least as far as mental health services are concerned. Speaking in broad terms, in 1985 service users were nowhere; in 2005 they are everywhere. Whereas service users were hardly involved directly in the development of the 1983 Mental Health Act, they have played an important role in de-bates around the current Mental Health Bill. It is unlikely, but not impossible, that any major development in the mental health field would now be undertaken without formal attempts to consult with people with direct experience.

The situation was very different in 1985. Mind and other voluntary organisations were 'the voice of the mentally-ill', speaking on their behalf without any coherent means of being sensitive to their true wishes. The few independent service user action groups that existed were unfunded, unappreciated and on the margins. When they did capture an audience they were accused of being extremists with nothing positive to offer.

Such sentiments would not be expressed today, at least not openly, and it is true to say that service users have now been recognised as rightful and valuable stakeholders in the process of developing better services. Service user activists have penetrated areas of the mental health system where their presence, let alone their positive contribution, would have been inconceivable 20 years ago. The fact that service users now run their own services, educate most groups of mental health workers, even provide a research team at the Institute of Psychiatry, the Service User Research Enterprise (SURE), is an indication of the different type of landscape we are now inhabiting. In short, people with a mental illness diagnosis have gone from being an absence to a presence in the mental health arena. Use of the descriptive term 'experts by experience' in recent years illustrates the distance that has already been travelled and hints at the potential that has still to be realised.

Drivers for change

It is an open question how much of this transformation can be attributed to service user action alone. There has been a steady demand for 'user involvement' from government and service providers and this has been vitally important both in stimulating the steady growth of action groups and shaping the types of activities they undertake. Frequently the necessity of finding service users to feed the system's need for consultation has been close to overwhelming. Service user groups have sometimes been created solely to meet this demand and it is not fanciful to suggest that if independent action groups did not exist, government would have to create something similar to replace them. So the demand for involvement has a life of its own and creates agendas over which service users may have limited control and which may not always serve their true interests. Having said that, there is no doubt that service user activists have profoundly influenced the way in which people with a mental illness diagnosis have begun to emerge from the shadows and be recognised as an important creative force in their own right.

Part of the success of service user action has been connected with the growing number of people willing to 'come out' and speak openly about living with mental distress. Challenging the secrecy surrounding this subject is essential to meaningful social inclusion and it is possible that such openness will eventually have widespread impact. At present, it is more likely that people will reveal their histories in and around mental health services and be less happy to speak out in other settings. There is even anecdotal evidence that some activists have become more cautious than they were in the latter respect as a result of persistent negative attitudes among the public. Despite the greater presence of people with direct experience in the media, stereotypes of dangerousness and 'alienness' are still prevalent and it is clear that progress remains frustratingly slow. Even so, the importance of mental health workers and service users 'coming out' should not be underestimated. Recent revelations by senior officers of the Royal College of Psychiatrists about their experience of mental distress would have been highly unlikely 20 years ago and illustrate the changes that are beginning to take place (Friedli, 2004a).

An important aspect of the development of action has been the growth of independent service user groups. These have formed the bedrock for activity, although it is important to recognise that work by activists on their own or within voluntary organisations for people with mental distress has also made a significant contribution. It was by no means inevitable that action would be focused around independent service user-led or service user only groups. In this respect, the fact that Survivors Speak Out, an organisation dedicated to support the formation of independent groups, was the first national network to be established was probably significant. Its existence helped ensure that new action did not become entirely directed through large voluntary organisations like Mind or the National Schizophrenia Fellowship (now Rethink).

The extent of the service user movement

It is difficult to be certain about the current number or character of service user action groups. The *On Our Own Terms* research report, (Wallcraft *et al.*, 2003) which covered England, developed a cleaned database of 896 groups. A recent article (Friedli, 2004b) suggests that there are 700 across the United Kingdom. There are problems in obtaining an accurate picture, partly as a result of the creation and disappearance of local groups, partly because it is not always easy to discover whether groups are service user-led, service user only or attached to voluntary groups. It is also true that people do not always use the same definitions to categorise them. These are interesting questions and important in any attempt to define a detailed description of what is going on. But in terms of providing a general picture of developments in the last 20 years, it is sufficient to say that there are now substantially more than 500 groups whereas in 1985 there were around a dozen.

From a base of about 50 groups at the end of the 1980s, growth in numbers accelerated through the 1990s. There can be little doubt that the NHS and Community Care Act 1990 (House of Commons, 1990) stimulated the formation of groups by requiring services to consult with their users. Statutory and voluntary organisations became more active in supporting service user action. User development workers began to be employed. Part of their brief was usually to establish forums through which the service user voice could be better heard. Funding, although not generous, was more available than in the previous decade. At the same time, service providers' requests for consultation had an effect on the character of action groups. Few felt strong enough to resist these requests even if they wanted to. The experience of being ignored or on the margins meant that involvement, on whatever terms, seemed too important to turn down. As a result, groups became more closely tied to the service system than groups in the 1980s that were more able to retain a separate position, offering criticisms and proposals from outside services.

The late 1980s and early 1990s also saw the establishment of a number of networking groups. These included the United Kingdom Advocacy Network (UKAN), the Scottish Users Network and the US-Network, covering Wales. Networks dealing with particular aspects of the service user experience became active, including the Hearing Voices Network and the National Self-Harm Network. The Manic Depression Fellowship became a service user-led organisation. During the 1990s, local groups set up by people from Black and ethnic minority communities also began to develop. On an international level, service users from the United Kingdom were involved in the creation of the European Network for Users and Survivors of Psychiatry. This level of activity was something different from what had gone before, albeit that some activists complained that action had lost its radical edge. Even so, the work in England of the Mental Health Task Force User Group (1992-1994) which collaborated with the Department of Health Mental Health Task Force to produce a number of important publications was seen as a significant success. The possibility of influencing policy at a national level, an opportunity that has not yet been properly realised, seemed quite realistic at that time.

The achievements of the movement

Before considering the types of action in which groups have become involved, and their successes and failures, it is worth noting the organisational achievements of the last 20 years of action. The successful existence of so many groups is witness to the way in which the activists' belief in the principles of self-organisation and self-help has been put into practical effect. Although some groups have been short-lived, many have been operating for ten years or more. The skills and long-term commitment required have been considerable and these are among the qualities which people with a mental illness diagnosis are popularly supposed to lack and be unable to acquire. Nevertheless, large numbers of activists, who at the time of their first involvement did not have organisational experience or expertise in collective working, have successfully acquired these skills. The fact that they have very often been working in small, under-funded organisations may actually make their achievement more remarkable. It is certainly not the case that keeping action groups up and running is an easy task and groups have had to come to terms with the ongoing mental distress of their members. Burn-out has been a feature. But these problems are not exclusive to service users. The creation and maintenance of action groups clearly demonstrates that the capacities of people with a mental illness diagnosis have been routinely underestimated. Sooner or later this revelation must penetrate mental health services and beyond.

Action has become very diverse and, as has already been suggested, service users have influenced most aspects of mental health services. These include: consultation and monitoring in connection with existing services and input into the development of new services; provision of training and education to all groups of mental health workers and involvement in selection of employees; undertaking service user-led research; creating and running service user-controlled services; and promoting new understandings of mental distress. Although local groups are unlikely to be involved in all these areas, most will be active in more than one. While action has always been largely concerned with mental health services, groups have also undertaken artistic activities and provided mental health awareness education to the general public. Work with the media has been an increasing concern.

Much of the contribution of service user activists has been made at a local level and there has been a limited amount of research detailing the impact of local action across the country. It seems likely that important but small-scale changes in the nature of services have been achieved rather than dramatic 'bricks and mortar' transformation. Attitude change and greater sensitivity and flexibility in the day-to-day running of local services have certainly begun to occur. Long-standing grassroots demands for independent advocacy and patients councils have also given service users more influence over their care and treatment and the environments in which they take place.

Obstacles to be overcome

It may be a cliché to suggest that while much progress has been made much more remains to be done, but there is a good deal of truth in such a generalisation. At this stage in the development of service user action there is a danger in being over-impressed, because of the low base from which action began. A number of obstacles continue to limit the service user contribution. These need to be acknowledged and overcome in the immediate future.

Credibility remains a crucial issue. In an evidence-based culture, evidence from service users frequently fails to measure up to 'scientific' standards.

The issue of representativeness has been a bugbear for action groups throughout the last 20 years and has never been tackled in an open way, allowing service providers to control when contributions from service users are taken seriously or not. The basis for such choices has usually not been made clear. Mental health professionals have regularly warned of the 'professional user', a slur which suggests that activists are not real service users and are not in contact with their constituency. It also betrays an anxiety and hostility around the fact that people with a mental illness diagnosis began to self-organise in a way professional groups have been doing for many years. By questioning the legitimacy of action in these ways, the establishment ensures that it remains in control.

As involvement has moved on from consultative work to other areas, concerns about credibility have continued. Service user-led monitoring and research (Rose, 2001; Mental Health Foundation, 2000) has often been undermined as not being 'real' research and lacking in scientific objectivity. The development of new understandings of aspects of mental distress like self-harm or hearing voices (Pembroke, 1994; Romme & Escher, 1993) has met with official scepticism for similar reasons. While consultation is a more acceptable, but still subtly controlled, activity, work in the above areas provides a far greater threat to the power base of the mental health establishment and so must be kept at arm's length. Despite the progress of the last 20 years, it is quite clear who is pulling the strings when it comes to the control of knowledge and understanding.

In view of this, it is not surprising that messages from people with direct experience take so long to have an impact. Mental health services grind extremely slowly. We are now in the midst of an epidemic of concern about acute care that has been intensifying since the late 1990s. Service user activists have been complaining about conditions on acute wards since the late 1980s (Good Practices in Mental Health/Camden Consortium, 1988). Suggestions about improvements and alternatives have been forthcoming over a similar period but have only latterly led to concrete results, for example ward round codes and crisis houses (*Openmind,* 2004; Mental Health Foundation/SCMH, 2002). Advance directives, now widely canvassed by professional and voluntary organisations in relation to a new Mental Health Act, were first taken seriously by service user action groups. In the mid-1990s, Survivors Speak Out was the first organisation to produce guidance for service users on writing their own advance directive. Without betraying too much bias, service users can claim to be providing many of the good new ideas in the above and other areas. Service providers' responses would benefit from some acceleration.

Resources are a major factor limiting the effectiveness of service user action. A great deal has been achieved on very little. While government and service providers' expectations and demands for input have steadily increased over the years, resources have usually not grown to match them. Although service user action groups are no different from other voluntary organisations in their dependence on unpaid work, there is a limit to the extent and quality of involvement that can be sustained without a greater commitment of resources. It is hard for activists not to detect the controlling arm of the establishment when it comes down to giving and denying money. Action has moved on in many ways and there are a much greater number of service users employed in the 'service user involvement industry' than there were in the 1980s and early 1990s (Snow, 2002). Nevertheless, there is a great imbalance between rhetoric and practice when it comes to funding. The service user contribution cannot be maintained, let alone developed, until this issue is successfully addressed.

The balance of power

Empowerment has become an important concept in recent years, particularly in regard to the lives of people who are long-term users of welfare state services. Apparently, mental health service users are becoming empowered. Like other fashionable concepts, partnership for example, empowerment can be used to soften or obscure realities as well as reveal them. Nevertheless, it is now so ubiquitous that it may be useful to look at the experience of people with a mental illness diagnosis in terms of their ability to control significant aspects of their lives.

Baldly stated, people with a mental illness diagnosis remain what they have always been: a fundamentally powerless group. While acknowledging that there have been recent improvements in their status, it is still clear that both in relation to mental health services and their position in society they reside somewhere near the bottom of the pile. The Disability Discrimination Act (1995), the Human Rights Act (1998) and the *National Service Framework for Mental Health* (DH, 1999) can with justification be called steps in a better direction. But they do not alter the basic reality. In 2005, people with a mental illness diagnosis are on the lowest rungs of the hierarchy of power. There are a number of factors that help ensure they will stay there for the foreseeable future.

Perhaps the most important of these is poverty, an issue that service user action groups could have done more to highlight in recent years. Poverty is a dominating feature in the lives of service users, robbing them of effective control of their destinies and diminishing the quality of day-to-day existence. Most of the experiences that cause mental distress are directly linked to a lack of money: poor housing, poor nutrition, lack of leisure opportunities, boredom, isolation and hopelessness. Many service users are unable to get out of the house and travel about locally unless they are lucky enough to have a free travel pass. A social existence of this nature cannot by the remotest stretch of the imagination be called empowering, no matter how much more involved service users are in their care and treatment. Looking back over the last 20 years and the increasing inequalities in British society, it is hard to feel optimistic that substantial changes are likely in this crucial area in the near future. Powerlessness linked to poverty is likely to remain a fundamental stumbling block.

Discrimination is another major obstacle to empowerment. While it is possible to argue that there is now more social awareness about 'mental health problems', public attitudes have not changed substantially. People may feel freer to talk, write or broadcast about a range of psychological problems. But psychosis is pretty much off limits and schizophrenia still fundamentally unspeakable. Since the public woke up to the reality that 'the mentally ill' were no longer being taken care of in the remote (in all senses) asylums, there is evidence that attitude change has been as much negative as positive. Certainly fear and preoccupation with perceived violence has increased. It is not clear that greater presence in the community has enabled people with a mental illness diagnosis to appear any less alien to the majority.

In some respects, everyone involved in the mental health field, service user activists included, may have been naive in hoping that somehow the best way of developing community care was to slip it in and hope that the community would not really notice. Perhaps the fact that the experts did not then know, and to an extent still do not know, how to effectively change public attitudes and behaviour had something to do with it. Whatever the reasons, people with a mental illness are still reduced to powerlessness through discrimination and denied any real equality of status. It invades every aspect of their lives. A survey of 778 service users (Read & Baker, 1996), which found that 47% had been abused and harassed in public and 26% had been forced to move home as a result of harassment, made the oppressive and tangible nature of discrimination very clear.

Mental health services have become more empowering. The opportunities for service users to influence their own care and treatment are greater now than 20 years ago. In this respect, the growth of independent advocacy, a steady development that owes much to the commitment of service user activists, has had a positive impact. Even so, there are still very basic shortcomings. Complaints about the amount and quality of talking and listening have not diminished. Service users still often feel they are not taken seriously or given sufficient information, particularly around medication. Respect and dignity are regularly demanded.

While the Department of Health claims that there is widespread satisfaction with services overall, numerous small scale surveys have revealed major disquiet among service users at aspects of the system. It does not seem impossible that satisfaction is linked to some extent to low expectations. At the same time, opportunities for individuals to become more involved are not always realised. Even after nearly 15 years, the Care Programme Approach, a significant step in putting service users at the centre of their care, does not seem to be operating effectively in parts of the country. Research evidence suggests that involvement in CPA, indeed even awareness of it, can be limited (Rose, 2001).

Any assessment of empowerment within services must take account of the Mental Health Act. On the face of it there are contradictions within a service that seeks to give its users more control over their lives and yet is prepared to exercise, increasingly, powers to detain and compulsorily treat them. The fact that this can happen legally, even when the individual retains the capacity to make treatment decisions, must be seen as an extreme form of personal disempowerment. Nor should its disempowering effects on people who are not detained under the Act but are potential detainees be underestimated. It is possible to see the Mental Health Act as a significant factor in the diminished status of people with a mental illness diagnosis.

Most service user activists have campaigned against any extension of compulsory powers. They have fought this issue consistently since the first proposals for Community Treatment Orders in the mid-1980s. Although they can claim some success in helping delay developments, it now seems almost certain that they will have to admit defeat and watch as the government increases its power to intervene in their lives and extend compulsory treatment powers into the community.

This is a significant rebuff to the beliefs underpinning the service user contribution in recent years, and in the eyes of many activists calls into question the sincerity of the current Government's commitment to empowerment and partnership. Moreover, it seems to confirm increasing suspicion that when it comes to the crunch, government will always respond more enthusiastically to the demand to control people with a mental illness diagnosis than to empower them. It is scant consolation that so many voluntary and professional organisations are now throwing in their lot with service user activists over the issue of compulsion.

Conclusion

From an activist's point of view the current period is a time of uncertainty – uncertainty about the future for service user action and about the future for people with a mental illness diagnosis as a whole. While life is more likely to be lived in the community rather than institutions, it is still far from clear on what terms that life will be lived or what its quality will be. On the one hand, the Government has recognised social exclusion as an issue and produced a useful report setting out ways of challenging it (SEU, 2004). On the other it seems content to go along with exaggerated fears of risk and dangerousness and tip mental health services further towards social control.

Even the recent growth of interest in creating employment opportunities has a darker side relating to the Government's desire to reduce the numbers of people with mental health problems on Incapacity Benefit. Already fears are growing that there will be greater commitment to decreasing overall benefit payments than to ensuring people are not shunted off into insecure and low-paid employment. At the same time, there is a continuing refusal to reward the contribution of service users on benefit towards the development of mental health services. In many respects, convincing signs that society is really interested in bringing any group of disabled people in from the margins are hard to find. The struggle for equal citizenship has a long way to go and it is not clear how well-equipped people with a mental illness diagnosis are to influence the outcome.

But, despite this, it is certain that service user action is not going to go away. A degree of permanence has been achieved and there are a number of challenges for the immediate future. One of the most important is to extend the involvement of minority groups in action. This is particularly relevant to Black and minority ethnic service users. Although there is a danger of underestimating their contribution in recent years, they have been under-represented in action and as a result their issues have not gained the priority they deserve.

Consideration also needs to be given to the type of alliances action groups establish. Much of the last 20 years has been devoted to work in collaboration with mental health professionals rather than other groups with similar experiences to service users. As issues to do with social inclusion and discrimination become more important there is an argument for developing alliances with other people with disabilities and other groups of welfare state users.

The demand for action is likely to continue because service providers will go on requiring 'user involvement' and because activists will want to open up other areas. Better organisation and co-ordination between groups will become more essential. There is an argument that a clearer ideology has become necessary to challenge biomedical orthodoxies that will always disempower. Certainly, it would be helpful if there was a clearer statement of shared beliefs and objectives. In the past many service user activists have been reluctant to create an overarching organisation that might claim to promote 'the service user voice' at a national level. This is beginning to change and a number of activists have been coming together to discuss setting up a broad forum that might increase the impact of action and develop a greater national presence. After 20 years, the issue of effectiveness has become particularly important.

Energy has never been a problem. Activists have been notably pragmatic up to now. Within mental health services there are a significant number of people, across all professional groups, who are willing to continue learning from the direct experience of people with a mental illness diagnosis. Services are more responsive. New understandings are being explored. Practice is starting to alter. In the next few years it will be interesting to see if activists can change services more radically while at the same time turning attention to a society largely untouched by service user action.

7 Primary Care and Mental Health

Alan Cohen

Introduction

To describe the development of primary care mental health since 1985 is to describe the development of primary care itself – and primary care has certainly developed.

Godber (1975) placed great emphasis on the role of general practice in the introduction of the NHS: "it was general practice, sustained by 37 years of National Health Insurance and gaining substantial additional support from the new system, which really carried the National Health Service at its inception".

Moon and North (2000) go on to say that in "successive Conservative and Labour visions of the NHS through the 80s and 90s... the therapeutic salience of general practice in the day-to-day operation of the NHS was matched by an increasingly central role in the development of the NHS as a party political project".

It is not surprising, given this perception of general practice as being at the centre of party political projects, that primary care has changed and developed.

The development of secondary mental health services, and the politics which have moulded the service we have today, have been subject to a quite different set of pressures: of managing people who are perceived to be dangerous (to themselves or others); of the stigma associated with mental illness; of the role of the user of the service as a participant in care; and of the apparent lack of competition within the internal NHS market. As a result of these pressures, the continuing priority of mental health services, as set out by government policy, is to provide care to people with a severe and enduring mental illness. The consequence of this is a gap in services, between very generalist primary care and very specialist mental health services. It is this gap that primary care mental health services have recently sought to bridge.

Over the last 20 years there have been few specific national policy documents relating to primary care mental health. It is only since 1999, in the *National Service Framework for Mental Health* (DH, 1999) that primary care services are specifically mentioned as having a role in providing care for people with mental health problems.

Prior to this date the way that primary care offered care to people with mental health problems derived from generic primary care policy, unlike specialist mental health services, which have been subject to numerous pieces of legislation and guidance.

The changing face of general practice

So what was primary care like 20 years ago? The GP contract at that time was a national contract, which paid a doctor according to the number of patients registered with them. There were incentives to deliver care, such as a per capita payment for childhood vaccinations or undertaking cervical cytology, and a number of increasingly idiosyncratic payments. One which was particularly well known and rarely claimed was a payment for arresting dental haemorrhage! None related to any form of mental illness. GPs employed their own staff, and worked from premises that they either rented or owned. Doctors themselves worked in a very similar fashion to the way that they work currently, providing a morning and afternoon surgery, with appointment slots. In the 1960s, the average length of an appointment was six minutes, in the 70s it rose to seven minutes, and then to eight minutes in the 80s, nine minutes in the 90s, and currently average consultation length is at least ten minutes.

Practices were starting to employ practice nurses, and to become more efficient through the use of practice administrators and practice managers.

The clinical work of primary care has remained unchanged, with the principle remaining that primary care, and specifically general practice, is the first point of contact for most people with any sort of health problem, and that general practice provides continuing personal care.

In the 1980s two seminal books significantly changed the way general practice, and more importantly general practitioners, perceived themselves. The first was called *The Future General Practitioner* published by the Royal College of General Practitioners (RCGP, 1972), which set out a direction of development for the profession. This direction was not just about career progression and premises development, but about the value and importance of the relationship between patient and doctor.

Written by a number of eminent thinkers in general practice, *The Future General Practitioner* described how this relationship influenced the presentation of symptoms, the understanding of those symptoms and the generation of solutions to health care problems. It encompassed not only the medical model of care, which focuses on diagnosing and treating illness, but its psychosocial aspects, such as the person's family life, their housing and their work. The impact of this book permeated all aspects of general practice, but in particular the newly created formal training programme for general practitioners (there had previously been no formal training for GPs). The consequence of this over the last

20 years has been a continuing 'love affair' with understanding, improving and analysing the consultation process, such that the membership examination of the Royal College of General Practitioners now has a compulsory element that requires the candidate to demonstrate excellent consultation skills.

The second seminal book for general practice was *The Doctor, the Patient, and the Illness* by Michael Balint (Balint, 1957). Although first published in 1957, this book has continued significantly to influence the way that general practitioners perceive their patients and hence themselves. Based on psychoanalytical principles the book allowed GPs to explore the relationship between GP and patient and to use that relationship to understand behaviour in both the consultation and in the wider environment.

Doctors who trained in the 1980s are now in the position of doing the training, agreeing the agenda, and delivering the new curriculum for GPs who are entering primary care today. The training that was received in the 1980s was so effective at providing a different way of looking at people's problems that general practice was fundamentally changed, but in such a quiet and, at the time, unremarkable way. General practice concentrated on understanding the bio-psychosocial background of the individual, concentrating on the person and their relationship with the GP, which mirrored the relationship between the patient and their wider environment. This individual approach was enormously attractive to professionals and to patients alike and as a consequence general practice grew in the public's estimation.

The impact of GP fundholding

However, the late 1980s and early 1990s saw a significant shift in national policy; the Conservative Government wished to use primary care services as a tool to change the NHS from a government-managed monopoly to a patient sensitive, market-driven organisation. The introduction of general practice fundholding in 1991 had a lasting impact on the way that care was delivered and on primary care mental health services.

The underlying principle behind GP fundholding was that a competitive market would drive quality up and prices down. An internal market should exist between purchasers of services (general practices and Family Practitioner Committees), and those who provided the care – the acute hospitals. General practitioners were given the resources: a single budget to purchase hospital activity and community services. Savings could be kept within the individual practice to further develop services.

For a branch of medicine that had previously concentrated on relationships, on understanding what wasn't said, the move towards a hard, uncompromising financial perspective in the way that care was provided, caused considerable heartache. The era of fundholding fundamentally changed primary care.

General practices now had to concentrate on practice management issues, financial accounting, delivering high quality care, and the primary-secondary care interface. So far as mental health services were concerned, there were some significant changes introduced.

Fundholding excluded the commissioning of services from specialist mental health hospitals. With the exception of thirteen pilot practices, the only way that fundholders could influence mental health commissioning was through the development of practice-based counselling services. (The phrase 'counselling' is used here not only to mean counselling itself, but also other forms of talking therapies provided by psychologists.)

Counselling was a service to which few practices had access prior to fundholding. Yet it was relatively cheap, and could be managed within the practice and by 1996 over half of fundholding practices had a counsellor working in their practice, compared to less than a third of non-fundholding practices. The presence of a counsellor also helped the GP to consider service re-design models. According to one popular rationale, if a GP were to refer a patient to a counsellor in practice, it might free up more time for the GP to see other patients. A second rationale was that if the patient had a psychological component to their need for specialist physical health care, introducing a counsellor to address those psychological needs might result in a saving in the costs of purchasing consultant care.

Whatever the reasoning, counselling in the early and mid 90s blossomed in primary care, with practices expecting counsellors to be part of the primary health care team, as much as a practice nurse or receptionist.

The development of counselling in primary care was rapid and, like any rapid development, went through a variety of stages. Initially there was the 'storming', and 'forming' stage, followed in the late 1990s by the 'norming' phase in which a professional representative body (the British Association for Counselling and Psychotherapy) was created to ensure counsellors in primary care were able to provide a professionally driven, clinically effective service. In the early days there had been concern about the rapid growth of counselling as there was no single nationally accepted qualification and anybody could set themselves up as counsellor. These counsellors were then unregulated and unable to demonstrate their clinical effectiveness in the same way as other professionals within the NHS.

Counsellors were frequently individuals who had contracts with general practices to provide a number of sessions per week. They were seen somehow as outside the NHS. The development of a professional body was welcomed as representing the 'coming of age' of counselling. With the Agenda for Change staffing reforms, introduced by the Department of Health in 2002, even counsellors are now, in 2004, having their job descriptions and terms and conditions reviewed, at last ensuring that they are considered to be part of the NHS.

Whilst fundholding may be considered by some as being responsible for many of the ills of the NHS, so far as primary care mental health was concerned, it was an opportunity to develop talking therapy services. It was a service that ran parallel to standard mental health services for people with severe and enduring mental health services; it was never really part of a comprehensive service.

To try to address this problem, thirteen general practice fundholding pilot sites were given a mental health budget to experiment with commissioning services for people with a severe and enduring mental illness. Although the practice sites had some limited success, it became clear that the principles of commissioning acute short term procedures did not apply to community mental health services. There are few practices in the UK sufficiently large to generate enough work for one complete community mental health team (CMHT). Most practices generate part of the workload of a CMHT, and for these practices each to commission a different type of service from a single CMHT raises important issues about equity and the ability of a CMHT to respond in different ways to different practices.

Analysis of the thirteen pilot sites also revealed that although individual practices might be able to influence the admission of patients to inpatient wards, by for example investing in enhanced services in the community, these were not able to generate any real savings for those practices as wards still continued to function normally: they still required staff on the ward, electricity and water etc. The pilots were not repeated. Some of the lessons learnt from these pilots are equally applicable now as primary care trusts start considering practice led commissioning (Cohen, 2004).

Labour's reforms of primary care

In 1997 the Labour Party won the general election and ushered in a new set of structures and principles for the NHS. Fundholding had been perceived, rightly or wrongly, to have contributed towards a 'postcode NHS' where services that were available depended on the postcode of the patient, rather than their clinical needs. The new Government introduced root and branch reform, which after eight years is still being implemented. Fundholding was abolished, and to ensure a consistent high quality service, national service frameworks were introduced for some areas of care. These frameworks set out the services and standards that had to be provided in all parts of the country, so that whether an individual was being treated in King's Cross, central London, or in rural Shropshire, the model of the service, and the standards, would be the same. The first *National Service Framework* (NSF) was published in 1999 (DH, 1999), and described the service that should be provided for people with mental health problems.

This *NSF* stated explicitly that people with a severe and enduring mental illness were the priority of the specialist mental health services. The *NSF* also set out seven standards for care, two of which related specifically to primary care (see Box 1).

Box 1: *National Service Framework for Mental Health* – standards two and three

Standard two

Any service user who contacts their primary health care team with a common mental health problem should:

❖ have their mental health needs identified and assessed

❖ be offered effective treatments, including referral to specialist services for further assessment, treatment and care if they require it.

Standard three

Any individual with a common mental health problem should:

❖ be able to make contact round the clock with the local services necessary to meet their needs and receive adequate care

❖ be able to use NHS Direct, as it develops, for first-level advice and referral on to specialist help lines or to local services.

(DH, 1999)

This was the first document published by any government of any political persuasion that explicitly set out the role of primary care to provide mental health services. Considering that 90% of people with mental health problems (including 30% of people with severe and enduring mental health problems) are managed entirely in primary care, this represented an important step forward. Although significant amounts of new money were allocated for *NSF* implementation, they were all directed at specialist mental health services. The standards relating to primary care had to be implemented from existing resources. Since there were many other changes in primary care at that time, not least the development of primary care groups and trusts, attention and resources were frequently directed else-where.

In 2000 the Department of Health published the *NHS Plan* (DH, 2000), a document that set out the further development and direction for the NHS. Within the *NHS Plan* was a section on primary care mental health, and the creation of a new worker – the Graduate Mental Health Worker. This represented a significant advance for primary care mental health. First, it acknowledged the role that primary care plays in supporting people with mental health problems, and secondly it identified a specific new allocation to develop and employ a new worker. The *NHS Plan* described the new worker thus:

> "One thousand new graduate primary care mental health workers, trained in brief therapy techniques of proven effectiveness, will be employed to help GPs manage and treat common mental health problems in all age groups, including children."

It is not the place of this paper to judge the effectiveness of these new workers, but to celebrate that at last the role of primary care in managing people with a common and enduring mental illness was recognised by the Department of Health.

Recent developments

In 2004, the Office of the Deputy Prime Minister published a report into social exclusion and mental health (SEU, 2004). This report was of enormous value for a number of reasons explored elsewhere in this book, but so far as primary care is concerned, it at last identified the extent of the disability that mental illness, common as well as severe, can have on individuals. The Social Exclusion Report identified that:

❖ 3 in 10 people of working age have sick leave in any one year due to mental illness.

❖ 91 million working days are lost due to mental illness.

❖ About one million people have been on long term sick leave due to mental illness and are receiving Incapacity Benefit (IB).

❖ Fewer than 10% are in contact with specialist mental health services.

❖ The proportion returning to employment, after having been on IB for 12 months or more, is less than 5%.

That so few of the people on disability benefits for mental health problems are in contact with specialist mental health services indicates that many are unlikely to have a severe and enduring mental illness: rather that they have common mental health problems that are managed entirely by primary care teams. The Social Exclusion Unit made many recommendations for implementation by primary care trusts that should, over the next years, have a significant impact on this group of individuals (SEU, 2004).

In 2003, the National Institute for Mental Health in England (NIMHE) developed a programme of mental health development that included a variety of work streams covering: the core skills of primary care professionals; the involvement of users and carers in developing and reviewing services in primary care; research; integrating care (and its link to the emerging new general practice contract); the commissioning of mental health services; and the development of the role of graduate mental health workers. The NIMHE Primary Care Board also developed a national primary care development programme that included the core skills educational programme, providing training for practitioners with a special interest in mental health, and supporting a national collaborative in common mental health conditions. The latter programme is to be run by the National Primary Care Development Team, and supported in part, by a grant from the Sainsbury Family Charitable Trusts.

In April 2004, a new national general practice contract was introduced. So far as primary care mental health is concerned, it is again to be celebrated that the contract acknowledged the workload that mental health issues present to the general practitioner. The contract addressed these issues through a number of different routes. It presented a quality and outcome framework for people with a severe and enduring mental illness, which gives practices financial incentives, for example, to improve the physical health care they offer this group, and by recommending a nationally enhanced service for depression. One of the benefits of the new General Medical Services contract (nGMS) was to describe what could be considered an "essential service", and that which could be considered "additional and enhanced services". These "enhanced services" for specific conditions came in the contract with a national tariff and a national specification. Whilst there may be criticisms of the details of aspects of the contract, it is nevertheless an important advance that these aspects of care were included.

In December 2004, the National Institute for Clinical Excellence (NICE) published guidelines on the management of depression and anxiety disorders (NICE, 2004). These guidelines, based firmly in primary care, describe best practice and make recommendations for assessment and treatment. Although these guidelines have only recently been published they are likely to have a significant impact on the way that care is provided.

Conclusion

The last eighteen months have seen a particularly significant focus on primary care mental health services. The *NSF* started this process by recognising the role that primary care plays. The *NHS Plan* took it further by creating a new role (the graduate worker) that should have a major impact on services. The Social Exclusion Report *Mental Health and Social Exclusion* (SEU, 2004) identified the extent of the discrimination and exclusion that people with mental health problems face, and reminded us that they are frequently not those in contact with specialist mental health services. NIMHE has developed and is implementing a national programme of primary care mental health development, and the implementation is supported by best practice from NICE guidelines for anxiety and depression. Finally the new GP contract provides a sound footing for incentives to support the effective development and implementation of these new services.

It is clear that over the last 20 years primary care mental health has come a long way, and in the last eighteen months has made significant advances to developing a rational and co-ordinated programme to improve services. These changes augur well for the future of primary care mental health.

8 Mental Health Teams
– Hitting the targets, missing the point?

Steve Onyett

Introduction

The last generation of team development has been associated with vigorous debate on teamworking in mental health services. Yet it is difficult to avoid the impression that some essential truths about teams have not been fully grasped. As we find ourselves at the half way point in the ten year plan set out by the *National Service Framework for Mental Health* (DH, 1999), it seems that teamworking in mental health has still to realise the contribution that it can make to improving the lives of users and the people who support them.

We have come a long way towards hitting the targets regarding teamworking in mental health. Those targets, most importantly those set in the *NHS Plan* (DH, 2000) the year after the *National Service Framework (NSF)* was published, have been based on sound re-search and experience. While this is welcome, there is also a danger of missing the point regarding teamworking in mental health. Two key points are being missed. The first is that teams, whether they be community mental health teams (CMHTs), crisis resolution teams, assertive outreach teams, or early intervention teams, are nonetheless teams and therefore subject to some well-researched factors that will promote or inhibit their effectiveness. The second is that the key function of teams is to promote and support *effective relationships* between service users and the people from their supportive social networks as the key means to developing valued outcomes. These people include family, friends and the team members themselves.

How did we get here?

The aims and features that should characterise the various types of teams that form part of the local service landscape are well described elsewhere (e.g. DH, 2001; Onyett, 2003). They have evolved in environments characterised by enduring failures to direct resources for effectively supporting implementation; by continuing problems in inter-agency working;

by mistrust of the policy agenda among influential professional staff; by public stigma of mental illness; and by a growing concern to manage the risk of service users harming themselves or others. There are many people who should be both very proud of what has been achieved and highly alert to the need to maintain improvement in an enduringly problematic and improvement-resistant environment (Rankin, 2004).

By the mid-1980s community mental health centres (as they were described then) had already begun to proliferate alongside the running-down and closure of large scale psychiatric hospitals. They promoted the shift of the centre of gravity for mental health services away from institutional settings to a more accessible local environment (McAusland, 1985). But to whom were they accessible?

It was at this time that community mental health centres were criticised for failing to serve people with the most severe and complex health and social care needs in the wake of similar findings in the US (Patmore & Weaver, 1991; Sayce *et al.*, 1991). The teams were criticised for being overly ambitious and unfocused in their attempts to offer a 'comprehensive' service. In practice this often meant offering a comparatively limited range of provision to a very broad range of people and failing to focus on those who were most in need of provision. Neglect of this group was further highlighted by evident shortfalls in investment in services for people leaving hospital and immense variations among local authorities in their expenditure on services for people with mental health problems (Audit Commission, 1986).

These problems were exacerbated by a lack of effective joint planning between health and social services, which in turn highlighted the need for 'case managers' with budgetary autonomy as a way of circumventing problems in inter-organisational collaboration. This role was later renamed 'care management' but was itself criticised for being resource-driven rather than needs-led, overly bureaucratic and for pulling social workers away from direct provision into more middle-management roles (e.g. Hudson, 1996).

It was about this time that commentators such as Peter Ryan at the Sainsbury Centre for Mental Health (SCMH) began to advocate a more practice-oriented interpretation of the case management role based on the 'strengths' model (Ford *et al.*, 1995; Onyett, 1992). This ideology foreshadowed much of the current focus on the 'recovery' approach with its emphasis on optimism, recognising the resources that users themselves bring, and the importance of relationships and social networks (NIMHE, 2005).

In 1991, the care programme approach (CPA) was introduced as the NHS's approach to planning personalised care in mental health. It followed from the first of several inquiries (the Spokes Report, DHSS, 1988) that served to undermine the public's confidence in community care. But CPA was seen by many as unhelpfully similar to the existing 'care management' approach being led by social services. This heightened the very problems in inter-agency working that it was meant to help resolve and so contributed to increased risk and poor planning.

Care management and the care programme approach were later effectively integrated, at least in policy guidance (NHS Executive/Social Services Inspectorate, 1999). Unfortunately this has not been reliably manifest in integrated care from a user perspective. With the integration of CPA and care management, the term 'care co-ordinator' was coined to locate the care planning function with one person who spanned health and social care. Many users still report not having a care plan or an identified care co-ordinator, let alone the copy of the care plan they were promised in the *NSF* (CHI, 2003).

Throughout the transitions from case management, care management and now care co-ordination, published guidance has shown a remarkable absence of references to these roles being undertaken in a team context, despite this being the reality of day-to-day practice. However, there has certainly been no lack of clear guidance on CPA implementation. Its history serves to illustrate the lack of leverage policymakers have on clinical behaviour unless they win hearts and minds round to a new way of working. We know from clinical experience how ineffective persuasion is in the absence of good quality information and respect for people's perspectives on the current situation (see the literature on motivational interviewing, e.g. Rollnick & Miller, 1995) yet we often fail to apply this knowledge when we relate to our colleagues.

In the early 1990s, a Sainsbury Centre for Mental Health survey of community mental health teams (Onyett *et al.*, 1994) highlighted the continued proliferation of teams and an improved focus on people with the most complex health and social care needs. But it also identified an enduring failure to seriously address the role and function of teams through a clear local planning process. Management of teams was seen to be comparatively weak. A study using the same methodology suggests that the situation has improved markedly since then, albeit with an enduring sense that more senior managers fail to provide enough support to the CMHT management role (McGuiness, 2004).

Fifteen years ago many services were already applying the learning from international experience and developing teams (often as government-funded demonstration projects) that were focused on specific client groups, with smaller caseloads and an emphasis on working with people in their own environments (e.g. Merson *et al.,* 1992; Dean *et al.,* 1993; Marks *et al.,* 1994). The *National Service Framework* in 1999 gave this the fillip it needed and brought with it a structure for performance management which included systematic service mapping of the reported numbers of teams in place year on year (for service mapping data see www.dur.ac.uk/service.mapping/amh).

Based on reports from 2003, in England there are now 260 assertive outreach teams (against a target of 220 by 2003), 174 crisis resolution teams (against a target of 335 by 2004) and 48 early intervention in psychosis teams (against a target of 50 by 2004). However, such comparative optimism does not always accord with reports from staff, users or carers who often find it difficult to reconcile what is reported centrally with their lived experience of the development of provision to meet local need (CHI, 2003).

For this reason, there are currently initiatives under way to survey systematically the development of crisis resolution, assertive outreach and early intervention teams as the basis for benchmarking and informed development work. It is only through getting these more detailed direct reports that the true state of local development can be systematically mapped. This information can also be used to support efforts to make transparent the funding coming through to support implementation. A recent survey of mental health service chief executives (*HSJ*, 2004) found that 60% were confident or very confident about meeting the *NHS Plan* (DH, 2000) targets for early intervention. For crisis resolution teams the figure was as high as 97%. Yet only 27% of chief executives were confident about their commissioners' ability to meet demand in the financial year and the same survey highlighted considerable anxieties about recruiting enough staff, particularly psychiatrists. There is thus a curious disparity between being confident about hitting the targets while simultaneously feeling ill-equipped to meet demand.

Banning the 'F word'

West *et al.* (1998) stated that, "Perhaps the major change in emphasis in research on teams in the last 15 years has been the shift from discussion of intragroup process to the impact of organisational context on the team". How the role of the team is defined within a local service system is of paramount importance. A study of the effectiveness of a wide range of health teams (of which 113 were CMHTs) found that unclear team objectives were the biggest contributors to poor functioning in a team (Borrill *et al.*, 2000). This was associated in turn with the absence of a clear team leader or co-ordinator or with conflict about leadership. They found better functioning teams had clearer objectives, higher levels of participation, a stronger commitment to quality, better support for innovation and improved mental health among team members.

There is no evidence of a magical synergy that makes people more effective simply by organising them into groups. Teams have to be designed with a clear purpose in mind. There is no reference to 'functional' teams (the much over-used 'F word' within mental health services) in either the *Mental Health Policy Implementation Guide* (DH, 2001) or the *NSF* (though 'functionalised' appears once). Yet the word has come to be used to differentiate the newer team models (crisis resolution, early intervention and assertive outreach) from (bog)standard CMHTs. This is part of the failure to see all these services as teams requiring premeditated design to be effective. If any team is not 'functional' it should not be running at all. Moreover it implies that CMHTs either have no function or are 'dys-functional'. While in some cases this may be true, the imperative is to consider how teams within a given locality work *together* to discharge the required functions collectively. These functions are well described by the *Mental Health Policy Implementation Guide (MH-PIG)* but the level of provision and its adaptation to local circumstances needs to be informed both by local needs assessment and positive practice (Chisholm & Ford, 2004)

Given the unambiguous targets and rigorous performance management that accompanied the development of the newer teams, it is interesting to note that the *NSF* in fact had a surprisingly permissive tone regarding service configuration. It stated that:

> *"CMHTs may provide the whole range of community-based services themselves, or be complemented by one or more teams providing specific functions. This latter model is most common in inner city and urban areas. Whichever model is used, the mental health system will need to provide the range of interventions and integration across all specialist services"* (DH, 1999).

The responsibility for being functional in this way lies with the whole local service system rather than the newer parts.

Mental health teams function within a complex environment typified by chronic lack of resources, poor information on met and unmet need, and multiple and often unmanaged and overwhelming demands from a variety of stakeholders. These include users and families seeking support and planners and policy makers investing teams with the role of promoting both social inclusion and social control. Achieving role clarity can often feel like a challenge.

There seems to be increasing experience in the field of open hostility between different teams serving the same patch. This is perhaps unsurprising. For existing services the introduction of the new teams has in some cases meant that they have lost staff and status while being expected to form the default service for those clients whom the newer teams either fail to take on or refer back for step-down care. The existing services therefore can find themselves in a situation of increasing demand, with depleted capacity and reduced control over their workload (Burns, 2004).

In this problematic context we need to find ways of getting team members to identify not only with their immediate team but with the work of the locality mental health service as a whole. West (2004) recently advocated that all local teams include in their objectives that they will act in a spirit of co-operation and altruism to other local teams. Achieving this is the task for leaders supported by effective processes for user participation, information systems that are fit-for-purpose and service improvement techniques that dramatically reveal the actual experience of local service users and their supports.

The General Secretary of the Royal College of Nursing recently observed that "Vision without action is hallucination" (Malone, 2004). Tried and tested modernisation techniques such as process mapping and plan-do-study-act groups can, with strong user and carer involvement, support these developments. But they need to be embedded in an effective *culture* of improvement for improvement to be a permanent part of the local landscape.

Making teams work

To qualify as a team at all there needs to be some level of interdependency between members to get a specific task done. One good principle of service design would be to think of the user as the central team member and then design the rest of the 'team' around them as a functioning unit where each player has a relevant task to perform.

The overriding condition for team effectiveness is clarity of aims. This is not necessarily an easy task. It requires clear leadership, good information, effective user and carer support and defended time to get it right. With support from the Leadership Centre, NIMHE is rolling out the Effective Teamworking and Leadership in Mental Health programme, a seven-day programme for 21 interdependent people within a given locality. The first two days of the programme focus on integrating the strategic (partly target-driven) aims of the team with a user and carer perspective on what is needed.

The programme then goes on to expose participants to the applied research that informs the design of teams. Some of this research runs counter to existing practice. Take for example the issue of size. As a complex decision-making unit, research would suggest that the optimal size of the team would be around seven, and that beyond around 10-12 its effectiveness is likely to be impaired. The challenge is to move from 'team' in name alone to 'real teams' that have: clear, shared, challenging objectives; the authority, autonomy and resources to get the job done; members who work closely and interdependently; clarity of team members' roles; a realistic size; and a positive team identity supported by effective leadership and clear operational management (West, 2004; Onyett, 2003).

The centrality of relationships

A desire to be more involved in decision-making was apparent in the first official survey of mental health service users last year (Healthcare Commission, 2004).

Placing users and their supports at the centre of team operation and improvement means that there should be at least one person within that team with whom the user feels they can establish a positive working relationship. The last 20 years have seen a powerful renaissance in the realisation that effective relationships between users and staff are the bedrock of local service provision. This is in no sense contradicted by the increasing use of coercion and a more explicit social control function for mental health services. Indeed it underlines the importance of defending effective relationships at all costs so that service users can exercise the most control possible over their lives and their involvement with services while also allowing them to depend on extra support when they need it.

Recovery is most effective when a holistic approach is considered that includes psychological, emotional, spiritual, physical and social needs. The NIMHE statement of recovery stresses the need to build trust, retain hope and work to involve families, partners and friends on the individual's own terms (NIMHE, 2005). Good quality enduring relationships are required to respond fully to an individual's expression of needs and preferences, particularly where there may be cultural differences between staff and service users. Making the best use of the diversity within teams and recognising that people will form stronger relationships with some team members than others can serve to support the development of shared understanding and agreement about ways forward.

Clearly, effective working relationships between staff and service users do not in themselves create good mental health services. They provide a necessary, if not a sufficient, condition for an environment in which users, their social networks and staff can work together to achieve the best outcomes given the prevailing conditions.

Sometimes establishing effective relationships in a team means that users need to be supported in working as far as possible with the team as a whole, as in assertive outreach, rather than just with identified individuals. This is often cited as providing a buffer against burnout for staff and a means of providing improved continuity of care (e.g. during staff absences due to holiday or sickness). However it also requires very strong communication within the team to ensure co-ordinated care that avoids duplication. In practice, teams appear to have taken a pragmatic approach to implementation that supports a team approach while also allowing users to exercise some choice about who they engage with and how (Chisholm & Ford, 2004).

What about the workers?

West (1994) considered team effectiveness to have three main components:

❖ **Task effectiveness:** the extent to which the team is successful in achieving its task-related objectives.

❖ **Mental health:** the well being, growth and development of team members.

❖ **Team viability:** the probability that the team will continue to work together and function effectively.

Teams are only likely to be viable over the long term if they are both effective in meeting their objectives and can attend to the well being of their members. While we should not neglect the key issues of staffing levels, pay and security, the key factor in keeping staff involved in the emotional labour of teamworking will be the *meaning* that they attach to their work. A Sainsbury Centre for Mental Health survey found that team members could be both emotionally exhausted and have high job satisfaction (Onyett *et al.*, 1995; 1997). This appeared to relate to the value that they and others attached to their work. Clinical contact with users was seen as a source of reward rather than as a source of pressure and the key sources of stress all related to issues that got in the way of being personally effective (e.g. workload, bureaucracy and lack of resources to meet clinical need).

Values are inextricable from the vision for a team's current and future operation. They state what is important, what the team stands for and the guiding principles that shape decision-making. Pendleton and King (2002) highlight a dramatic decline in morale and motivation among providers of health care and attribute this largely to staff being asked to work in ways that interfere with or compromise the values that they hold most dear. Perhaps the most oft-cited example of this is the view expressed by staff that their managers are so concerned with risk management that they feel held back in supporting users to take creative and appropriate risks to promote their independence. A new Mental Health Act that is perceived as overly concerned with social control may exacerbate this problem.

Clever (1999) was moved to seek a "call to renew" values based upon key touchstones such as excellence, kindness, integrity and loving relationships. West (2004) described the challenge of improving the morale and effectiveness of the workforce as helping staff achieve clarity about what they should be doing, and creating environments in which they felt valued, supported and respected. He described the role of leaders as "to create organisations that are basically kind". Here again SCMH and NIMHE are set to play a key role in making the issues of values and the mental models that people deploy in their work a more explicit focus of training and development (NIMHE, 2004).

Community teams in 2005: threats and opportunities

The Mental Health Policy Implementation Guide stated that:

> "CMHTs, in some places known as Primary Care Liaison Teams, will continue to be a mainstay of the system. CMHTs have an important, indeed integral, role to play in supporting service users and families in community settings. They should provide the core around which newer service elements are developed. The responsibilities of CMHTs may change over time with the advent of new services, however they will retain an important role. They, alongside primary care, will provide the key source of referrals to the newer teams. They will also continue to care for the majority of people with mental illness in the community" (DH, 2001).

CMHTs may have an increasingly important role in promoting equitable access. Corry *et al.* (2004) highlighted concerns from the voluntary sector that the implicit emphasis in new models of working (such as assertive outreach and early intervention) on younger people is increasing the risk that older people with longer term problems become even more vulnerable to loneliness, isolation and a poor quality of life.

Community teams have a central role in promoting the social inclusion of people living these more marginalised lives, and in doing so they work in close collaboration with primary care, families and other helping agencies. SCMH provides some useful guidance on practical steps that teams can take to promote more socially inclusive practice. They include:

❖ Ensuring that users of the service and the team itself have good access to expert benefits advice, for example by working in partnership with an independent welfare rights agency or organising an outreach advisor service from Jobcentre Plus (SCMH, 2004a).

❖ Understanding and maximising all opportunities to take up paid employment, e.g. through 'Permitted work' and managing the risk of triggering an inappropriately timed medical review (SCMH, 2004a).

❖ Ensuring that staff are fully briefed on the role and function of 'Supporting People' services, and providing them with practical support in order to promote the tenure and appropriate housing and support of service users (SCMH, 2004b).

New legislation may make the role of community mental health staff in maintaining public confidence in community care more explicit as they become the agents of community supervision. This could have a profound and damaging effect on the meaning that staff attach to their work. No matter what the values in play, coercive practice will inevitably be influenced by the allocation and adequacy of resources for service provision. Coercion tends to increase when effective community interventions are not available (Diamond, 1996). Where coercion becomes applied as a short-term solution to long-term problems concerning lack of resources, services become crisis-driven, overly concerned with social control and delivered in a manner that precludes the development of good quality relationships and collaborative work with service users.

Social control may not be a new feature of mental health services. However, it still behoves us to exercise that role in the best way possible in the interests of service users and their supports. This means locating as much power and control with users as possible. Perkins and Goddard (2004) highlight that user involvement in the management of mental health services is associated with more effective engagement in care, which is itself associated with reduced risk. Inquiries into homicides and suicides, events that are tragic for anyone with a stake in effective community care, consistently highlight the simple need to ensure that users have enough time and support from staff to feel understood and to avoid isolation and loss of hope. This is clearly not promoted by a crisis-driven, coercive approach to provision that is not based upon users' own preferences and aspirations.

Community teams continue to be subject to a range of seemingly contradictory pressures, including an urge towards a greater emphasis on social control while simultaneously promoting social inclusion and fair access. Working effectively with these tensions at a local level requires that we are more explicit about the values and practices in action. *The Ten Essential Shared Capabilities* (NIMHE, 2004) provide a helpful platform for achieving this. Local improvement will also require that we take into account both the structure of local services and the processes that take service users and their supporters into them – sometimes to the exclusion of other more helpful opportunities.

Alongside structure and process we also need to be mindful of the importance of local organisational culture and the different cultures pervading different parts of the local system. Working across parts of the system can help with this, for example through specialist mental health staff working within primary care settings. In this case it is important that community teams do not attempt to colonise and reform the primary care culture but rather to integrate with it and exploit its strengths. For example, there is evidence that users and their supports value primary care specifically because it works with them over longer periods, sees them within their normal social context and operates models of understanding mental health that are less diagnostically and individually-focused (Rogers & Pilgrim, 1993).

Conclusion: focusing on what works

I have not attempted the definitive review of whether teams in their various forms have been effective over the past 20 years. Sashidharan *et al.* (1999) alerted us to the fact early in these debates that research is far from neutral or disinterested. He asserted from his perspective as an experienced clinician that it would be mere common sense to expect more intensive and targeted community services to make a positive difference to users and their supports. The challenges lie in how we implement these improved services.

Despite the inevitable shortcomings of current research knowledge it is possible to conclude that where teams are intensive, proactive and centred on developing good working relationships with users they can effectively engage them, keep them out of hospital and in many cases improve important aspects of their lives. However, in order to be economically viable the intensity of provision needs to achieve a threshold where it becomes a valued alternative to inpatient care for people with severe mental health problems. Field experience is illuminating the sort of local adaptations that can be made to local circumstances (Chisholm & Ford, 2004; Onyett, 2003).

What has also emerged over the past 20 years is that the 'soft' stuff of leadership, team and organisational culture, of staff values and attitudes and of relationships between staff and users and their supports are likely to be just as important in improving the experience of service users as the 'hard' stuff of caseload size and the specifics of team operation. While these key aspects of design remain important, we should still be mindful of the wider cultural changes that have occurred in how organisational life is now understood. This reflects a shift away from technical solutions based on engineering metaphors and top-level driven management to insights based upon understanding of complex, local systems that (like any system in nature) are self organising, locally evolving and often surprising in the way change and the dispersal of good ideas and positive practices happen. As Malone (2004) commented, if we are to achieve more than just change and aim for a positive transformation, "we need to develop a taste for chaos".

Achieving change in this context means moving beyond team 'awaydays' and uni-disciplinary training that fails to include exposure to both the research and the lived reality of teamworking. It requires a stronger emphasis on those shared values and practices that span disciplines, and stronger recognition of the importance of local organisational culture. Whole systems thinking emphasises the need to make conscious and to develop shared values, purposes and practices within and between organisations and their members. It requires that we bring together the perspectives of a wide range of people across the full range of services for people with mental health problems (Iles & Sutherland, 2001).

Mental health services are characterised by tensions between strongly competing interests and imperatives. These need to be made more explicit if the values of service users are to be brought to bear on decision-making and to create a shared view of what needs to be done. Community teams need to be increasingly accountable to users. They should be planned around their needs and aspirations, user-led in implementation and thus ultimately more effective in achieving user-valued outcomes. This will not only help service users but have the enormous added benefit of restoring meaning to the working lives of those people involved in supporting them.

9 The Social Context for Mental Health

Elizabeth Gale and Bob Grove

> *"Mental health care does not take place in a vacuum. It influences, and is influenced by, the society in which it is practised."* (Ion & Beer, 2003)

Over the past 20 years there have been many changes in mental health practice relating to the provision of more holistic services, the prevention of mental health problems, the understanding of the risk factors which increase the prevalence of mental ill health, and the promotion of mental health as a positive concept. Mental health is now a priority area not only at the Department of Health but also within the Department for Education and Skills, the Department of Work and Pensions and the Office of the Deputy Prime Minister, as it relates to social exclusion and regeneration. Mental health is no longer seen solely as a health issue but as a cross-cutting theme of interest for real joined-up thinkers.

To deliver services effectively it is essential that those commissioning, providing and evaluating health care and health improvement recognise the social, economic and political environments in which they practise, and the impact these environments have on the overall health and well being of individuals and communities.

Mental health is dependent on people's social environment, experiences, age and family situation. The existence of mental health problems, and the terms, concepts and language we use to describe them, have been contested areas of debate for decades. There have been many arguments that mental health is a construction of social context and that the inter-linking relationship between an individual's social experiences and health is difficult to define and deconstruct.

One example of this inter-linking would be the relationship between deprivation and health. Social deprivation and isolation increase a person's risk of developing mental health problems. Conversely, people with mental health problems are more likely to suffer from social deprivation and exclusion – they may be unable to work, possibly leading to losing their home, they may be unable to maintain social relationships, they may be discriminated against – because of their mental health problems. Social status has a direct impact on health status and vice versa.

The importance of the social context for mental health has expanded over the last two decades in three main ways.

Firstly, there has been a recognition of the importance of social contact and participation, and the impact of exclusion and isolation on an individual's mental health and well being, whether or not they are currently diagnosed with a mental health problem.

Secondly, levels of stigma related to mental health problems and the discrimination which people with mental health problems so often experience individually and collectively, have remained largely unchanged but are now recognised as being detrimental and worth tackling.

Finally, mental health promotion and the enhancement of public mental health are becoming embedded in other broader agendas such as tackling health inequalities, improving the social environment for health and well being and enhancing the mental health of the nation.

This chapter looks at the way the social context for mental health has changed, or endured, in some key areas over the past 20 years.

Exclusion and isolation

It has long been recognised that adults with mental health problems are among the most excluded and disenfranchised groups in society. Mental health problems can be both a cause and a consequence of social exclusion. In recent years the recognition of the impact of the social world on health and well being has increased, culminating in the report of the Social Exclusion Unit in 2004 (SEU, 2004).

Unemployment rates are high among people with mental health problems. Only 24% of adults with long term mental health problems are in work. This is the lowest employment rate for any of the main groups of disabled people (Office of National Statistics, 2003). People with mental health problems are far more likely to lack financial security; they are nearly three times more likely to be in debt (Meltzer et al., 2003) and more than twice as likely to have problems managing money as the general population. They may be excluded from financial services due to their diagnosis – up to a quarter of people with mental health problems are refused these services (Read & Baker, 1996). Many people with mental health problems experience homelessness and housing problems which can exacerbate their ill health and inhibit their participation in local communities (SEU, 1998).

It is clear that mental health problems lead to social isolation and exclusion and that these experiences often exacerbate an individual's poor health and well being. The charity Mind recently estimated that over 84% of people with mental health problems feel socially isolated compared with 29% of the general population (Mind, 2004). People with a severe mental health problem are three times more likely to be divorced than those without a diagnosis, and are less likely to have established social support networks or to be members of social clubs, even though they wish to participate more actively in their local communities (Meltzer *et al.,* 2003).

Social contact is known to promote good mental health and to help people with mental health problems to recover, as well as bringing an overall improvement in quality of life. Good personal support networks, for example friendship or a confiding relationship, and opportunities for social and physical activities, protect mental health and enable people of any age to recover from stressful life events like bereavement or financial problems (Cooper *et al.,* 1999). Access to information and practical help can play an important role in reducing feelings of exclusion and isolation.

People with a small primary support group of three people or less are at greatest risk of mental health problems (Brugha *et al.,* 1993), while social support reduces death rates and susceptibility to infection and depression, notably in older people (Cohen, 1997; Oxman *et al.,* 1992).

Social exclusion does not only have an impact on the health of individuals. It also has an impact on whole communities by destroying social capital. Levels of trust, tolerance and participation – all important measures of social capital – are now widely recognised as critical factors in determining health (Wilkinson, 1996, 2000; Cooper *et al.*, 1999, Kawachi *et al.*, 1997, Kawachi & Kennedy, 1999). One study, indeed, found that while a person's trust in their community was related to their mental well being, trust in friends and family was not (Berry, 2000).

Evidence that civic engagement and levels of participation may be more important for health than other elements of social capital have further strengthened interest in community empowerment and the reduction of social exclusion (Campbell *et al.,* 1999). There is a robust case for addressing social fragmentation and obstacles that stand in the way of community participation by excluded groups, including people with mental health problems. (Campbell & McLean, 2002)

From segregation to citizenship

In the past 20 years there has been a move from care in institutions to appropriate care in the community. In more recent years this has focused on working directly to achieve social inclusion and citizenship for people with mental health problems, rather than simply relocating segregated services into community settings and hoping that this will promote acceptance and reintegration (Bates, 2002).

This shift in attitudes and thinking – which is still incomplete – can be illustrated by looking at what was happening for mental health service users in 1985 in life domains such as work, housing, leisure and education, and comparing it with the best of what is happening now.

In 1985 most employment services were still located in protected settings, either on the sites of large mental hospitals or in nearby industrial or commercial buildings. Although much valued by people who attended 'industrial therapy', the move into ordinary employment from these settings was very low (Boardman, 2002) and for most people with severe and enduring mental health problems waged work was considered too demanding.

By 2005 evidence had piled up indicating that most service users want to work (Secker *et al.,* 2001) – at least part time – and that individual placement and support services can dramatically improve the numbers of people finding and maintaining open employment (Bond *et al.,* 1997). In the United States, researchers compared the employment rates of those who used day services and those whose day services converted into supported employment services. They found that the proportion of people moving into employment from day centres remained around 5% (the same as for the old sheltered workshops), while numbers from day centres converting to supported employment rose to between 15 and 35% (Becker *et al.,* 2001).

The latest service developments are concerned as much with preventing people losing their jobs as with helping them get back to work from long term unemployment (Thomas *et al.,* 2003). This can help to avoid the spiral of ill health and unemployment from beginning in the first place.

Current thinking about housing also shows a shift towards supporting people in ordinary housing. In the 1970s and 1980s, the emphasis was on creating 'halfway houses' and 'group homes' which assumed that people with mental health problems required protected settings which they shared with other service users and which were convenient for staff to manage.

Progressive services in 2005 not only encompass home care and treatment, but are piloting Shared Ownership Schemes (e.g. Advance Housing, 2004) and experimenting with Direct Payments to enable tenants with support needs to employ their own support workers. The Supporting People funding scheme is proving particularly helpful as a means of promoting independent living (SCMH, 2004).

In education, arts and leisure activities the same shifts in thinking are apparent. The move is away from creating alternative settings in which service users are in the community but not part of it, towards providing "bridge builders" (SEU, 2004) who help people engage with the same services, clubs and facilities as other citizens. A journal called *A life in the day* (published by Pavilion since 1997) has charted and celebrated the great burst of energy and creativity released by this new paradigm in which supporting people to lead the kind of lives they want, rather than merely alleviating distress and preventing harm, is seen as the main objective of services.

Supporting people to undertake their personal journey to a better life – 'recovery' – also implies a different type of relationship with professionals. In the new paradigm professionals are not seen as providers of rehabilitation so much as facilitators who create the conditions in which people can empower themselves. Twenty years ago, mental health services were moving from institutions to the community – but service users remained separate from the people who lived around them. Now, service users themselves are becoming members of those communities.

Such a shift in thinking and power relationships is not easy for people trained in a more traditional way to take on board, and the new paradigm is a long way from being embedded within all mental health services (Seebohm *et al.,* 2002). However, the direction of travel is becoming clearer with every year that passes. It is now commonly accepted that it is no use waiting for stigma and discrimination to be eradicated before embarking on inclusion, but rather that successful, practical community bridge building and citizenship initiatives are an essential part of the process of challenging society to reassess its relationship with those it regards as mentally (and sometimes dangerously) ill.

The last 20 years has seen a major move from care in institutions to care in the community. Until recently, inclusion has been about gaining the public's acceptance of services in the community; more recently it has focused also on inclusion of the service users themselves in their communities.

Stigma and discrimination

People with mental health problems consistently identify stigma and discrimination as major barriers to health, welfare and quality of life (Dunn, 1999; DH, 2001; Mental Health Foundation, 2000; Sayce, 2000; Rethink, 2003). Stigmatising beliefs, and the discriminatory practice they legitimise, lead to the exclusion, isolation and social injustice which people with mental health problems experience regularly.

Conventionally, stigma has been understood as a relationship between characteristics of a person and socially constructed negative stereotypes (Goffman, 1963, Jones *et al.,* 1984).

Discrimination is defined by the United Nations as the less favourable treatment of persons. This treatment can limit an individual's or group's rights to opportunities, often due to attributed rather than actual characteristics. Understanding the beliefs that justify discriminatory behaviour is considered to be essential to identifying appropriate ways in which to challenge such beliefs.

Much work has been completed in the last decade on the causes of stigma and discrimination, as well as the evidence which underpins effective practice in challenging it internationally.

The relationship between attitude (such as prejudice) and behaviour (such as discrimination) is complex. One should not assume that one automatically leads to the other or is due to the other. For example, people can be prejudiced but act fairly, and people can discriminate unintentionally. Much depends on the specifics of the situation: how socially acceptable discrimination is; whether there are any costs or penalties involved; and if there is any surveillance or cause for redress.

Over the last 20 years, many programmes have aimed to increase awareness, reduce stigma and challenge discrimination around mental health issues. Campaigns and programmes have been managed by the Department of Health, the Health Education Authority, the Royal College of Psychiatrists, Mind and many others. Yet attitudinal surveys by the Department of Health (DH, 2003) and the reviews of discrimination by the Disability Rights Commission show that change is slow in coming, if indeed it has come at all.

A review of changing public attitudes in the 1990s showed that mental health/mental illness was difficult to define and no single term adequately described it for all groups (DH, 1999a). Levels of awareness of mental illness had grown throughout the 1990s and it was increasingly viewed as 'normal'. This has led to a polarisation of views. Certain diagnoses, for example those linked to life events such as post natal depression, became more acceptable. On the other end of the scale severe and enduring mental health problems remain strongly stigmatised and are generally considered to be shameful, and people with such diagnoses are still feared and disliked.

Overall, tolerance towards people with mental health problems appears to be declining and the roles in society they are allowed to take are those with minimal responsibility and which minimise perceived potential harm. The stereotypes they still face include: moral taint, linking mental illness with evil; the 'life not worth living view'; the supposed hopelessness of having a life-long mental illness; and the meaningless of the opinions of the 'mad', discrediting the views and voices of people with mental health problems as unworthy by their very nature (Sayce, 2003).

Programmes to tackle mental health stigma now place more of an emphasis on discrimination and action than on stigma and attitudes. This approach redirects the focus of programmes onto perpetrators of stigmatising behaviour and away from its victims (Sayce, 2000) and has proven to be more successful in other countries running national mental health programmes. Such programmes have gone a long way to deepening our understanding of what works in this area (Gale *et al.*, 2004).

Sayce (2003) identifies our need to challenge discrimination in four ways:

❖ Legally, by using rights based legislation such as the Disability Discrimination Act;

❖ In public debate, by increasing the visibility and audibility of people with mental health problems and reducing the social distance considered to be between 'us' and 'them';

❖ By challenging the direct and indirect impact of discrimination, changing the public's hearts and minds;

❖ By ensuring that tackling discrimination and social exclusion are included in other policies, for example by placing a positive approach to employing people with mental health problems in policies around recruitment and retention among employers.

These are not mutually exclusive approaches: they are inter-dependent and they require the development of partnerships outside the mental health sector and indeed outside the health and social care sector altogether to deliver them effectively.

In 2004, the National Institute for Mental Health in England (NIMHE) released a five-year strategic plan to tackle stigma and discrimination on mental health grounds, entitled *From Here to Equality* (NIMHE, 2004). The plan is in response to the Social Exclusion Unit report (SEU, 2004) and its implementation is supported across Government. The plan outlines the programme's vision to enable people of all ages who have or are affected by mental health problems to live as equal citizens. It aims to focus less on the 'wrongs', such as stigma and discrimination, and more on the 'rights' – the rights of people with mental health problems not to be discriminated against in any part of their lives. This is the largest investment ever made in relation to the reduction of stigma and discrimination.

Broader agendas

The final element of the changing perception of mental health is its inclusion within broader agendas related to health and social care, well being and renewal. Since 1997, there has been an official recognition of the importance of inequalities on health. In 1998, the government-commissioned Acheson report clearly showed the differences between the health of the rich and the poor and set the agenda for narrowing them (Acheson, 1998). One of the most disadvantaged groups, as has already been stated, are people with mental health problems, who have poorer overall health than the general population. Therefore the increase in the relevance of and the investment in the reduction of inequalities in health has in part included programmes aiming to improve the health status of people with mental health problems.

The inequalities targets in the *NHS Plan* (DH, 2000) have required those working in health and social care services to engage with and involve more the local communities they serve. Colleagues working in urban renewal, regeneration and local government are also being tasked with considering and addressing the psychological and emotional impact of deprivation and exclusion on communities. Mental health and well being is being increasingly considered relevant to community regeneration, enhanced empowerment and the social fabric of society. This should make quality of life indicators that measure the impact of how people feel a legitimate tool for assessing progress, and in some areas a legitimate outcome of regeneration and renewal.

The *NHS Plan* also outlined the importance of involving the public and the patients who use the NHS. This agenda is not about structures; it is about a cultural change required to ensure that consultation is real, that views are considered, and that suggestions are taken forward to improve the reach and the relevance of the NHS. Patient Advice and Liaison Services (PALS) and Patient and Public Involvement Forums will provide the mechanics for delivering enhanced involvement and participation, with resulting health benefits.

Health promotion and community development programmes have also become more 'mainstreamed' into broader policies within specific settings. For example those who are interested in health at work do not now consider mental health at work programmes to be related simply to recruiting or indeed retaining people with mental health problems in the workplace but also to supporting and promoting the mental health of all employees within an organisation. Similarly, mental health programmes in schools are not solely the responsibility of special educational needs co-ordinators or about children with behavioural problems. They are part of broader 'Healthy Schools' programmes ensuring that the emotional health and well being of young people is being seen as key to their development and their future achievements (Lister-Sharp *et al.*, 1999).

Some advances are considered to have taken place through the increased commissioning of voluntary sector agencies in service provision. Agencies which in the past have been seen as on the outskirts of health policy are now far more central to the development, delivery and assessment of services in some areas.

Mental health promotion is enshrined in Standard One of the *National Service Framework for Mental Health* (DH, 1996b). England is the first country in Europe to have a standard in health policy related solely to the promotion of mental health. National service frameworks concentrating on older people, and on children, also explicitly mention the promotion of mental health as an important outcome. This is to be welcomed. However, concerns have been raised about the lack of support for mental health promotion and the need to build capacity and support sustainability in these fields.

Public health has also increased its profile recently and mental health is now included more centrally in public health policies than ever before. The Treasury-commissioned Wanless reports considering the future of public health were criticised for ignoring the underpinning nature of mental health and well being. Although mental health was recognised as one aspect of health and well being, discussion was limited to unhealthy lifestyle choices among people with mental health problems (Wanless 2004; Gale & Greatley, 2004).

The concept of public mental health has been undervalued and largely ignored within broader public health and mental health circles over the past decade. Public health debate has focused largely on the individual and the individual's ultimate responsibility for their health and their lifestyle choices. Yet the idea that individuals can be fully engaged through improved information, support for positive decision making and the promotion of healthy lifestyles is naïve.

However, its time has come. Positively, and most recently, the publication of the public health white paper *Choosing Health: Making healthy choices easier* includes mental health as one of six underpinning themes. The paper states that mental well being is now considered to be crucial to good physical health and to making healthy choices (DH, 2004).

Public mental health is the science and art of preventing disease, prolonging life and promoting health, both physical and mental, through the organised efforts and informed choices of society, organisations, public and private communities and individuals. The evidence for promoting public mental health is growing and the contribution this discipline can make to a range of outcomes is clear. It can prevent suicide, reduce relapse, aid recovery, enhance mental health literacy, improve self esteem and self image, strengthen life and coping skills, increase social support, reduce social exclusion and isolation, increase social capital and improve quality of life.

Another change in the past decade is the development of new evidence for public health. The development of the TREND statement (transparent reporting of evaluations with non-randomised designs) is one important attempt to broaden the range of approaches to finding out what works in public health practice. Evidence bases are moving towards acknowledging the breadth of what constitutes effective practice in the improvement of public health, which can only encourage the debate and the development of indicators to improve public mental health as well.

Poverty and lack of opportunity are not simply related to economic disadvantage but also to social, educational, environmental and cultural disadvantage. The new agenda for public mental health should relate to participation and redistributing real opportunities. The past 20 years has proven to us that improvements can be made in relation to mental health and its measurement and the delivery of its promotion through a range of different agendas.

Active citizenship, social cohesion and social justice are key to improving health for everyone. The future points us to concentrating on enhancing social inclusion and opportunities for participation, not solely on reducing levels of exclusion; on supporting the human rights and civil liberties of people with mental health problems, not solely on reducing stigma and discrimination in specific settings; and on promoting the public's mental health through the full range of public services.

10 Social Inequalities and Mental Health
— An integrative approach

Jennie Williams and Frank Keating

Introduction

This chapter draws together work exploring the significance of social inequalities for mental health and mental health services; work that has gained impetus and status over the last 20 years. At the beginning of the new millennium the importance of inequality is finally being acknowledged in the public agenda of mental health services (see, for example Acheson, 1998; DH, 2002, 2005; NIMHE, 2003), though these policy directives and initiatives are only just beginning to make their mark on service provision. While increasing numbers of people within mental health services recognise the importance of social inequalities, most are very uncertain about what this means for their practice. Against this background, our intention is to make the developments in this disparate field as meaningful and as accessible as possible to practitioners.

Defining social inequality

So what is social inequality? It exists when attributes such as gender, 'race' and class affect our access to socially valued resources including money, status and power – our chances of having lives of comparative privilege or disadvantage. These arrangements are unfair because they serve some groups at the expense of others: there are fundamental conflicts of interest at their core. However, inequalities are often difficult to detect and challenge because they are hidden by ideologies that name the processes associated with their perpetuation as 'normal' and 'just', and their damaging consequences the fault of the disadvantaged. In short, we are discouraged and deflected from thinking about inequality, and even when we make an effort it is generally much easier to have conversations about diversity, multiculturalism, social exclusion and difference.

Reflecting on social inequality is also personally challenging, because it is an invitation to review our own lives i.e. our own experiences of advantage, disadvantage, power and powerlessness. Not only does the current arrangement accord privileges and disadvantages to each of us, but it also provides the basis for our many identities. When we ask "Who am I?" and "Who are you?", it is gender, 'race' and ethnicity, class, age, sexuality and so on, that come to the fore, accompanied by a sense of how these characteristics are valued or devalued and their capacity to shape access to good things in life. It is common, therefore, to encounter both social and personal resistance to the process of thinking and talking about social inequalities. Not only is there resistance, but the structures in which mental health professionals work do not provide 'safe spaces' to talk about these issues (SCMH, 2002). The question therefore remains: how can we progress the discourse on inequalities and mental health if we are not able to talk about it openly?

Mental health providers need to be alert to the major determinants of inequality in this society, which include, gender, 'race', class, age, and sexuality. They also need to be especially mindful of the power relationship between those who provide and those who use mental health services and the disempowering consequences of being labelled a user of psychiatric services. Inequality becomes additionally significant for the majority of people who use mental health services because it is both a cause and a consequence of their distress. The recent report by the Social Exclusion Unit (2004) found that people with mental health problems are amongst one of the most disadvantaged and socially excluded groups in society; this is cogently illustrated by Trivedi (2002) in her account of the "spiral of oppression".

Arguably, some dimensions are likely to have greater psychological significance than others. Gender inequality has particular significance for mental health because families are the place in which females and males whose structural relationship is one of inequality live together, and where we construct our gender identities as children and adults. That said, in practice we caution against leaping to conclusions about the significance of any particular parameter of a person's life: there are no short cuts to hearing from them about their lives (Kalikhat, 2004). It is also important to remember that while some dimensions of social inequality such as marital status are not major determinants of social structure they may nonetheless be of great psychological significance for particular individuals, and mental health workers need to remain open to this possibility. The individual's own narrative and lived experience should be at the core of any attempt to understand and respond to the impact of social inequality on their physical and emotional well being.

Status of the approach

People engaged in struggles for equality and civil rights have largely been responsible for bringing the psychological consequences of inequality to the attention of the field of mental health. Theory and practice have emerged in the context of social movements representing the interests of women, people from Black and minority ethnic communities, gays and lesbians, and mental health service users. This has two important implications.

Firstly, literatures have typically developed along one dimension of inequality with a focus on the implications for the disadvantaged group. As Beckett and Macey (2001) observe, "academics, policy makers and activists in Britain have a long tradition of ignoring the intersections and interactions between these social divisions", though there are some scholars who are an exception to this (Beckett & Macey, 2001; Weber, 1998; Williams, 2005). To illustrate, the recent policy aimed at improving service provision to people from Black and minority ethnic communities (NIMHE, 2003) contains no mention of gender. Keating et al. (2003), in a review of mental health services on issues of ethnic diversity, found that a potent mix of gender blindness and negative views of minority cultures contributes to Black and minority ethnic women's mental health needs being severely neglected across the spectrum of research, policy development, service provision and practice. Such unitary definitions of oppression have limited value within mental health services; they limit our perception of the complexity of human existence and also create situations that force different groups to compete for resources.

Secondly, achievements in the development of knowledge and service provision that give centrality to inequality lie mainly at the margins: this is nicely illustrated by the title of the women's mental health strategy *Into the Mainstream* (DH, 2002). The limited impact is also evident in mainstream policy makers' and service providers' attempts to address inequality. These are typically located in the context of discussions about service access or inequalities in health outcomes – limited debates that are premised on the uncritical acceptance of the status quo within mental health services: particularly the traditional processes used to categorise, name, and treat emotional distress. The thinly scattered service developments that do take social inequalities seriously are typically characterised by their struggles for survival, recognition and acceptance. By definition these small scale specialist services to groups such as women and Black and minority ethnic groups offer a perspective that involves an understanding of the reality of people's experiences in the context of social inequalities (Keating, 2002). However, the knowledge and competencies accrued within these services are seldom integrated into mainstream practices, nor do they inform the training of mental health professionals (Scott & Williams, 2004).

In summary, the body of knowledge about the implications of social inequalities for the field of mental health which has accrued during the lifetime of the Sainsbury Centre for Mental Health (SCMH) lacks both integration and value. Given this we suggest that important next steps are to develop an integrative framework that will enable mental health practitioners to respond sensitively and constructively to the complex effects of social inequalities.

Inequalities and mental health

A common approach in this field is to trawl the research literature and statistical data to look for differences in mental health outcomes for people from different social groups defined by gender, race, and so on. However, interpreting this kind of data is notoriously tricky as evidenced by the long and troubled debate about 'race', culture and schizophrenia (Fernando, 2003). Instead, we suggest it is more constructive to take the existence of social inequalities as a factual starting point and from this explore the implications for mental health and mental health services. Once this decision has been taken it is not difficult to find out about the mental health implications of social inequalities.

These are some of the ways of building the knowledge, wisdom and skills to work from an inequalities perspective:

❖ Listening to, and continuously learning from, those who know most about the challenges of psychological survival in an unequal and unjust society, as well as the risks of revictimisation within mental health services.

❖ Becoming familiar with the facts and figures outlining the parameters of people's lives in this inequitable society; these are readily available on government websites as well as those posted by campaigning and advocacy groups (see References).

❖ Becoming knowledgeable about the extensive body of work exploring the mental health impacts of inequalities (Ballou & Brown, 2002; Belle & Doucet, 2003; Bhui, 2002: Fernando, 2003; Rogers & Pilgrim, 2003; Tew, 2005; Williams, 2005).

❖ Becoming knowledgeable about theory and research that sensitises us to the ways that the power of psychiatry can support the interests of privilege to the detriment of the individuals it seeks to help (Burstow, 1992; Fernando, 2003; Penfold & Walker, 1984; Rogers & Pligrim, 2003; Williams, 1999).

❖ Selectively using 'grey' literature and the media (e.g. *Asylum* magazine; *What Women Want,* Mental Health Media, 2002).

❖ Reflecting on our own experience of power and powerlessness.

❖ Seeking information about innovative services (Mental Health Media, 2002; Rivera, 2002).

❖ Getting involved in relevant social action (Cogan, 1996).

Developing understanding

The crucial areas of concern for mental health practitioners and policy makers are mapped out below, along with brief commentary. Our intention is to inform the development and provision of training, and to support self-directed learning in the absence of institutional support. It is important to state at the outset that Figure 1 draws attention to the damaging *potential* of social inequalities and invites us to think respectfully about the dynamic ways in which people resist, struggle and cope: it is not a description of inevitable consequences for individuals or indeed for mental health services.

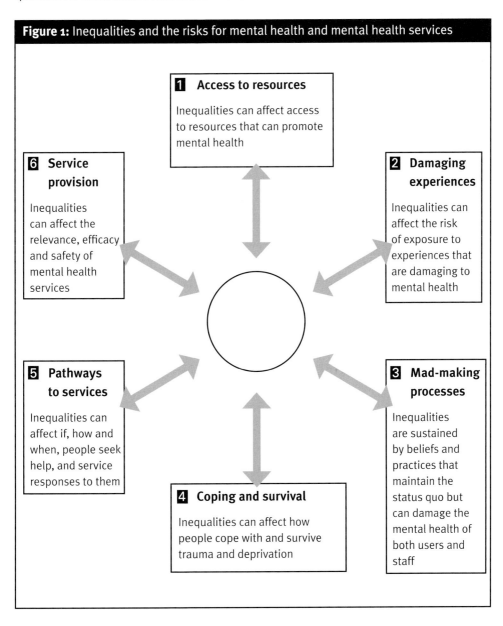

Figure 1: Inequalities and the risks for mental health and mental health services

1 Access to resources

Inequalities can affect access to resources that can promote mental health

6 Service provision

Inequalities can affect the relevance, efficacy and safety of mental health services

2 Damaging experiences

Inequalities can affect the risk of exposure to experiences that are damaging to mental health

5 Pathways to services

Inequalities can affect if, how and when, people seek help, and service responses to them

4 Coping and survival

Inequalities can affect how people cope with and survive trauma and deprivation

3 Mad-making processes

Inequalities are sustained by beliefs and practices that maintain the status quo but can damage the mental health of both users and staff

1. Access to resources

Social inequalities create conditions under which some groups of people are treated less favourably than others in society, including having less access to resources known to support and promote psychological well being. These resources include satisfying work, money, education, leisure, housing, status and value. For example, the latest census (White, 2002) found that people from minority ethnic groups had far higher rates of un-employment than their white counterparts. In addition to the wealth of statistics and research findings that can be used to broaden our understanding of these parameters of people's lives, we need to listen carefully to lived experience. To illustrate, this is Alison, 31, who earns the national minimum wage of £4.50 an hour.

> "Equality doesn't exist in my world. I'm working in a 21st-century sweatshop for the minimum wage with hundreds of other women. All our managers and supervisors are men, who show us no respect or consideration. Is this what equality was supposed to be about? All the crappy jobs in this country are done by women like me, who also do most of the child-caring. Having it all's a joke – we have the worst of all worlds." (quoted in Appleyard, 2004)

The effects of social inequalities on access to material, social and psychological resources is typically detrimental to people from disadvantaged social groups. However, it is important for mental health workers to be aware that these conditions have the potential to strengthen relationships within groups which enable people to seek support and vali-dation from each other. The power of these processes in achieving social and personal change are well documented (DeChant, 1996).

2. Exposure to damaging experiences

Social inequalities create conditions which increase the likelihood that some groups of people will be exposed to experiences that are detrimental to their mental health. These experiences include working in de-valued, dangerous and unpaid jobs, and being exposed to bullying, harassment, abuse and violence. For example, we know that offences are committed against people simply on the basis of their membership of a minority group:

> "To be attacked, beaten up or otherwise abused, and to find the police re-sponse one of indifference, is the not infrequent experience of homosexuals, and blacks too ..." (Pyke, 2004)

The 2000 British Crime Survey estimated the number of racially motivated offences against minority ethnic groups at 280,000 (Clancy et al., 2001). Furthermore there is evidence that crimes motivated by hatred are particularly damaging to psychological well being (White, 2002). There is also an extensive literature on the challenges to psychological well being from domestic violence and sexual abuse (Williams, 2005) and racial oppres-sion (Fernando, 2003; Trivedi, 2002). It is crucial for the quality of mental health services that staff have the competencies to help people come to terms with such experiences in ways that enable them to claim a better future.

3. Mad-making processes

Systems of inequality are given stability by a range of social psychological processes, some of which have particular significance for mental health.

Identity

A significant part of our identity is derived from our membership of social groups, and we receive greatest encouragement to adopt identities that are compatible with the requirements of the social status quo. Hence, people from disadvantaged groups are expected to possess or acquire qualities that are useful to those who are more powerful; and to be grateful and compliant despite their oppression. To illustrate, 'good women' are not expected to get angry, and disabled people are expected to be co-operative and grateful. The psychological significance of such requirements and injunctions are of central significance for mental health (Burstow, 1992; Williams, 2005).

The mental health costs of inequalities are not only borne by the disadvantaged but also by those who are privileged by the status quo: there are mental health risks when identities are derived from unequal relationships. To illustrate, masculinity underpins the social dominance of men; being manly is equated with power – over women or other men – but this is at the cost of emotional entitlement. Successful male socialisation requires men to be silent and strong, leaving individuals little scope to acknowledge and deal constructively with feelings of vulnerability or powerlessness.

> *"As a boy I was not allowed to feel scared...if I cried or broke down I was a sissy not a man. My father was lost at sea when I was nine years' old. I was informed...that I was now the man of the house, had to be strong, keep my chin up and look after the women...the forced denial of the experience of grief was impossible for me to cope with"* (quoted in Bertram, 2003).

Furthermore it is white, middle-class heterosexual men, who are most likely to accrue the rewards of fulfilling this script. This is unlikely to be the case for men who are poor, unemployed, from Black and minority ethnic communities, for whom the gap between the expectation of dominance and their experience of powerlessness may be extremely distressing.

Significant dynamics

It is crucial for mental health service providers and policy makers to be sensitive and responsive to the ideologies, processes and practices that maintain and challenge inequalities. These dynamics are detectable in our own lives, in the lives of people using mental health services, and in the interactions that take place throughout mental health services. The evidence base for their existence and effects is scattered throughout the various inequality literatures. While most of this literature is concerned with risks to the mental health of the disadvantaged, there is also growing evidence about the risks to the mental health of people from privileged social groups. Though this latter development does not have much appeal to the activists who have developed this field, it is important to remember that those people who use mental health services are most likely to be the casualties of systems of inequality rather than those who have reaped their material and psychological benefits. Table 1 (opposite) shows some of the dynamics that can help develop a systemic understanding of the personal damage and distress created by inequalities.

4. Coping and survival

We can draw on many resources in our struggles to survive and cope with the damaging effects of inequality including religion, spirituality, attachment to communities, social networks and political action (Faulkner & Layzell, 2000). However, our access to the internal and external resources that help us survive the losses and challenges of life is also affected by social inequalities (Waldrop & Resick, 2004; Walters & Charles, 1997). The internal factors include self-esteem and identity derived from, for example, our gender, 'race', and class; the external factors include social support, money, education, time and community involvement. Hence the survival strategies of people whose lives are shaped by multiple oppressions – which may include reliance on self-medication with alcohol or drugs, eating distress, and self harm – need to be understood in the context of severely limited options, and a likely background of repeated failure to change their lives and feelings. Most mental health workers have not been trained to appreciate this, and in the absence of these understandings the strategies used by individuals to survive intolerable feelings often evoke alarm and punishment and keep the focus on problems, rather than understanding and respect, and an acknowledgement of the individual's own coping strategies and resilience (Williams *et al.*, 2004).

5. Pathways to services

Research confirms that gender, 'race', class and sexuality are significant determinants of an individual's pathway to, exclusion from and avoidance of services. A social inequalities perspective is crucial for making sense of these patterns and for taking steps to address problems of equal access. It provides an important reminder that attempts to address inequality in access should not be narrowly associated with an increase in services. As Rogers and Pilgrim (2003) note it is crucially important to take heed of the social control functions of mental health services. A stark illustration of this is the over-representation of African-Caribbean patients in the most controlling sectors of mental health services (Fernando, 2003; SCMH, 2002). Their entry into care is characterised by hospital admissions under a section of the Mental Health Act, over-involvement of the police, the forcible administration of medication and contentious staff-user interactions (Goater *et al.*, 1999; Thornicroft *et al.*, 1999). Within these communities there is understandable reluctance to engage with mental health services which are associated with being detained in hospital in confined and restrictive environments, and the risk of death (SCMH, 2002). On the basis of this evidence it is clear that the priority should be to challenge inequalities within mental health services, while promoting the development of services that are responsive to the mental health implications of sexism, racism and other inequalities.

Table 1: Significant dynamics			
Practices & Processes	**Function**	**Risks for the mental health of the disadvantaged**	**Risks for the mental health of the advantaged**
Attribution of inferiority and superiority *"I was classed as no good 'cause I was a single parent."* (quoted in ReSisters, 2002)	Supports the status quo in inequitable relationships	Damage to sense of self; limits control over one's body and labour, and access to resources	Anxiety, anger and frustration at not actually feeling powerful and invulnerable; risks to self and others of attempting to take more power and control; contact with criminal justice system
Blaming, derogating, ridiculing *"But that's what these men do... they make you feel so small that you agree that everything is your fault."* (quoted in Humphreys & Thiara, 2003) *"I was told that I encouraged the other patients."* (quoted in Baker, 2000)	Supports inequality by identifying a person or group as the problem not inequality	Damage to identity and self-esteem; self doubt; feelings of embarrassment, guilt, sadness and depression; of being harmed not helped by mental health services	Erodes the hope and creativity of mental health staff and increases their risk of burnout
Denial and indifference *"Doctors don't want to know about past domestic violence, just up the valium and I was walking around like a zombie."* (quoted in Barron, 2004) *"No action was taken and I was told 'as I am good looking' I should expect it to happen."* (quoted in Baker, 2000)	Supports inequalities by denying, minimising and trivialising their consequences	Isolation, vulnerability, increased risk of further abuse; of being harmed not helped by mental health services	Alienation and dehumanisation of mental health staff
Deference *"You know so much more than I do; so tell me, what should I do?"* (quoted in Burstow, 1992)	Supports inequalities by giving power and authority to others	Internalisation of feelings of inferiority; loss of power and control and associated risk that this will be abused; acceptance of psychiatric authority	Overburdened with feelings of responsibility for others; limited feedback from others can impede personal development

Table 1: Significant dynamics *(continued)*

Practices & Processes	Function	Risks for the mental health of the disadvantaged	Risks for the mental health of the advantaged
Discrimination *"I went to see a psychiatric nurse who was assessing me. She was completely homophobic...she was so rude to me and so horrible to me...and I was very, very vulnerable and I thought I just can't face it."* (quoted in King & McKeown, 2003) *"Coming to this country [from Jamaica]...working and working to bring up your family and every day being treated like that, people looking down at you."* (quoted in ReSisters, 2002)	Maintains and accentuates existing inequalities, may be unconscious or conscious	Blocks opportunities; limits access to valued resources; increases exposure to conditions that are damaging Denigrating views may be internalised with implications for self validation and social support Fear of seeking help from services	Can erode self-respect and personal integrity
Exploitation and abuse *"The psychiatric problems have stemmed from the way I was treated as a child – physically abused by my mother, sexually abused when I was 10, raped when I was in care at 13, raped by other males in care when I was a bit older."* (quoted in ReSisters, 2002)	Validates and takes advantage of an inequality – this can also occur in the context of provider/user relationships in mental health services	Damage to sense of self; dissociation; alienation; chronic exhaustion	Alienation from meaningful intimacy
Intimidation and coercion	Use of fear to preserve existing power relations	Erosion of self; feelings of fear and of being trapped and helpless	Alienation from meaningful intimacy
Legitimation and authorisation	Supports inequality on grounds of normality	Having experiences and distress labelled as madness and being treated chemically	
Marginalisation *"Women's mental health issues appear to have a lower status and services rely heavily on professionals having a personal interest."* (quoted in Williams et al., 2001)	Supports inequality by limiting power of disadvantaged groups	Not being heard or taken seriously	

Table 1: Significant dynamics *(continued)*			
Practices & Processes	**Function**	**Risks for the mental health of the disadvantaged**	**Risks for the mental health of the advantaged**
Medicalisation and individuation *"Our needs are ignored, we are treated as illnesses."* (quoted in Williams *et al.*, 2001)	Supports inequality by identifying a person or group as the problem not inequality	Decreases chances of recovery Increases chances of experiencing further oppression and trauma	Burnout amongst staff
Normalisation *"Pathologising women who do not follow gender norms in lifestyle/behaviour..."* (Williams *et al.*, 2001)	Validates inequality and punishes deviance; normalises abuses of power	Punitive reactions to 'social deviants'	Constrains personal development and expression of vulnerability – limits ways of coping
Objectification (sexualisation, racialisation etc.) *"When I was in the 4th grade [at the crippled children's school], a man began to trap me in the hall and say sexual things as well as touch me inappropriately."* (quoted in Nosek *et al.*, 2001)	Power advantage embedded in inequalities are used to exploit the least powerful	Poor self image; self-blame; risk of exposure to traumatic experience These experiences can be intensified within psychiatric services (Cohen, 1994; Keating, 2002: Williams, 2005)	False sense of entitlement; Alienation from meaningful intimacy
Projection *"Klein's theories about projection, where an individual projects his/her own intolerable feelings onto the other are central to an understanding of the relationship between bully and target."* (Martin, 2004)	Power advantage embedded in inequalities used to get rid of unwanted feeling	Justification for male violence Resentful and demoralised staff can displace feeling on to patients	Detrimental to self development and the possibility of genuinely caring about people
Resistance, challenge and change *"When people are pushed hard and when they're treated in a brutally unjust way, the reaction is sometimes the opposite of what you might expect. Sometimes the worm turns."* (Pyke, 2004)	People from disadvantaged groups survive by being knowledgeable about the workings of the more powerful – in some conditions this leads to collective action	Can lead to personal empowerment	An opportunity for personal and moral development i.e. to come to terms with the past and to take responsibility for our behaviour

6. Service provision

Dominant models of distress which emphasise diagnosis, individual pathology and medicalised responses to distress, serve the status quo by detracting attention from social inequalities. In these ways, the connections between a person's behaviour, distress and lived experience are severed, and without these understandings behaviour is easily understood as meaningless, out of control and dangerous. Treatments and interventions continue to be based on narrow clinical definitions which result in a medical response with a reliance on prescribing medication, even though many mental health practitioners are now well aware of the psychological damage caused by the abuse and misuse of power, injustice and maltreatment (Rogers & Pilgrim 2003; Williams & Scott, 2002). It is simply that in the absence of relevant training staff are at a loss about how to respond.

Mental health services replicate the discrimination experienced in wider society, which includes an over reliance on the more controlling and restricting aspects of treatment. Here, a service user talks about her experience of seeking help from mental health services as a Black person:

> "...coming to mental health services was like the last straw...you come to services disempowered already, they strip you of your dignity...you become the dregs of society" (quoted in SCMH, 2002).

Gender and other social inequalities also have discernible effects on understandings and definitions of mental health. To illustrate, even though femininity is demonstrably linked to clear mental health risks, studies find that women who have internalised feminine characteristics are generally considered to be normal and mentally healthy. Furthermore, as we have noted elsewhere (Williams & Keating, 2000) when training desensitises mental health workers to the powerful effects of inequality on mental health, they are unlikely to be aware of the potential damage inherent in inequalities within services. This is evidenced by the tolerance shown towards abuse and violence within mental health services. It also includes the failure to understand the power relations associated with the huge inequality that exists between providers and users of services. The effects of this are extensively reported by service users (e.g. ReSisters, 2002) who complain of being endlessly judged and found wanting; of being blamed for not changing or for being difficult, angry, and fearful; and who describe being devalued and treated disrespectfully and having their needs, reputations, histories and futures defined by others.

> "Nobody treats you like a human being, you are treated like another commodity...and yet you will have to go through dissecting a lot of your personal issues and it goes nowhere...why is it that professionals treat us like second class citizens, especially within mental health ...why is it that you can never erase a label? Why does it stick for life?" (quoted in SCMH, 2002)

People known to use mental health services are likely to be further burdened by being categorised in such ways (Rogers & Pilgrim, 2003). For example, a brief spell in hospital can seriously affect an individual's access to their children, social networks, employment, and stable accommodation.

Conclusion

The mental health workforce needs a thorough-going understanding of the implications of social inequalities. For this to be achieved there needs to be a much greater willingness to give inequality priority on the mental health agenda, and for it to be a central theme in the training of all mental health staff. When this happens staff are empowered (Scott & Williams, 2004), so it is encouraging, therefore, that 'Challenging Inequality' has been identified as one of the *Ten Essential Shared Capabilities* (NIMHE, 2004) that all staff are expected to have. It seems that the NHS modernisation and equalities agendas, however imperfectly realised, are providing some opportunities for change.

One of the important ways in which mental health services can respond at this point is by a clear commitment to the principles and values that underpin drives toward equality. It is also absolutely crucial that social inequalities are identified as having central significance for mental health and service provision. Inequalities, and their impact on the language, organisation and practices of mental health services, should not go unchallenged. This means incorporating an integrated understanding of different oppression systems into our thinking, and developing a shared approach to exploring the implications for services. It also means avoiding simple allocation of blame and responsibility, and the application of neat divides between victims/perpetrators and user/providers of mental health services. There is now a powerful case for a radical change and we can no longer plead ignorance as an excuse.

Acknowledgement

Many thanks to the people who provided helpful comments on the earlier draft of this chapter, especially Premila Trivedi.

11 A View from Abroad
– A new vision of stewardship

Howard H. Goldman

There is a long tradition of foreign commentary in which visitors from abroad write about the institutions of other lands. Herodotus, the Father of History, travelled the ancient world of the 5th century BC to write the first histories of wars and social practices in the golden age of Greece. During the first century AD, Josephus moved from his birthplace in Jerusalem to Rome and described military battles and life in the ancient capital of the Empire. Alexis de Tocqueville from France, and Charles Dickens each visited the United States in the mid-19th century and wrote of the emerging nation and its social organisations. In particular Dickens commented on asylums and other social welfare institutions that were first established during this period.

Special insight is often attributed to foreign visitors, who are thought to be able to see what natives are unable to discern. I do not subscribe to this theory of special insight. More likely the observations of foreign visitors provide a slightly different perspective. I am pleased to have the opportunity to provide a view from America and to extend the tradition of foreign commentary on the occasion of the 20th anniversary of the Sainsbury Centre for Mental Health (SCMH).

This chapter presents some observations from 20 enjoyable and informative years of collaboration and travelling "across the pond". I review several similarities and differences between mental health services in the US and the UK with a special focus on the role of mental health authorities and the evolving nature of stewardship for mental health services.

Similarities between the UK and the US

Mental health is fundamental to health and social welfare

Although stigma and discrimination frequently characterise attitudes and behaviour toward individuals who experience mental health problems and the whole field of mental health, there is a growing understanding that mental health is fundamental to health and social welfare. In the US, this view was embodied in both *The Report of the Surgeon General* (DHHS, 1999) and in *Achieving the Promise,* the final report of the President's New Freedom Commission on Mental Health (DHHS, 2003). In the UK, this view is reflected in official documents, such as *The National Service Framework for Mental Health* (DH, 1999) and the Sainsbury Centre for Mental Health's *Working for Inclusion* (Bates, 2001).

The notion that mental health is fundamental to health and social welfare is associated with the growing recognition that *recovery* from a mental disorder is not only possible but is to be expected (DHHS, 2003; SEU, 2004). Even if not achieved fully, recovery is an appropriate goal – individuals who experience a mental health problem should be able to go to school, to work and to participate in the community. Of course, while in both countries recovery is a goal and attitude change an expectation, in reality neither is routine practice. Stigma and discrimination persist and mental health is still easily marginalised and separated from the mainstream of general health and social welfare concerns and policies.

Treatments for mental disorders are effective, but associated social problems remain

Mental disorders and the wider range of mental health problems are complex health and social welfare problems with broad implications for participation in society. In spite of growing awareness of this complexity, mental health policies in both countries still emphasise the medical elements of treatment, and do not provide sufficient support for the social welfare aspects of care. For example, medication and psychotherapy services are more common practice than supported employment and supported housing. As a consequence, people with mental health problems are "better, but not well", as they receive more care than ever before but still fall short of complete recovery and full participation in society (Glied & Frank, forthcoming). A new emphasis on recovery and social inclusion means that services increasingly focus on more than just symptoms. They target social, educational and occupational functioning, adequate housing, reduced involvement with the criminal justice system, and improved quality of life. Scientific advances provide an evidence-base for optimism, but practice in the US and UK does not match the promise of more effective services (DHHS, 1999; DH, 2003). There is a gap between needs and services and between potential and actual quality of care. And these disparities do not fall randomly in the population of either country.

Culture, race, and ethnicity – as well as poverty – magnify the disparities

Cultural diversity has become the rule in the US and the UK. 'Minorities' have become 'majorities' – or certainly pluralities – in some local jurisdictions, and 'culture counts' in the design of good mental health services. This perspective on mental health policy is reflected in both the *Supplement to the Report of the Surgeon General on Culture, Race, and Ethnicity* (DHHS, 2001) and in the Sainsbury Centre for Mental Health's report *Breaking the Circles of Fear* (SCMH, 2002), and the subsequent initiative. Members of cultural and ethnic minorities, as well as people who are poor, are more likely to experience certain mental health problems, to receive fewer of the services they need, and to receive services of lesser quality. They also experience worse outcomes when they *do* receive services.

Fragmentation plagues the mental health service system

There is dysfunctional separation among important elements of the mental health service systems in both the US and the UK. Fragmentation makes it difficult to meet the complex needs of individuals with enduring mental health problems, when services are needed from general health and social welfare systems as well as from specialist mental health providers. Public and voluntary organisations and different levels of government also differ widely in terms of responsibility and accountability. Both countries recognise that better integration is needed in service delivery, policy development and programme enactment. Services and supports from diverse agencies within the human service system must be orchestrated to meet the complex, fundamental needs of individuals with mental health problems and to reduce service disparities (DHHS, 1999, 2003; DH, 1998a, 1998b).

Differences between the UK and the US

What are rights to care in the UK are privileges in the US

Although service users and providers face similar clinical and social problems in both countries, health services are a right for all citizens in the UK. These services, as well as housing and income replacement, are not rights but privileges in the US, where about 45 million people have no health insurance (Kaiser Family Foundation, 2004) and where a much smaller proportion of the Gross Domestic Product is spent on transfer payments for disabled individuals than in the UK (Mashaw & Reno, 1996). In consequence of these policies, service programmes in the US have fewer options for supports and services than their counterparts in the UK. On the one hand, this deficiency has spurred innovation in the US in terms of mental health service programmes providing directly for these basic needs. On the other hand, this need for innovation distracts clinicians from treatment and other specialised service provision.

The UK is deservedly proud of its National Health Service (NHS) and its local authorities with respect to their commitment to serve the needs of the whole population. Care is not ideal in either country. Resource scarcity in the NHS results in priority setting, targeting services, and cutting surgical waiting lists (SCMH, 2003). In some local US communities, individuals with enduring mental health problems may fare better than their UK counterparts, but the overall quality of life for people with mental health problems may be better in the UK.

Variety and choice of services is greater in the US

It is my impression that there are many more types of services for people with mental health problems in the US compared to the UK. That is true for professional as well as service user-led programmes. Within service types there are also many different ways to deliver that treatment or service. For example, a psychiatric rehabilitation programme in the US might offer pre-vocational training, supported employment services, or employment within the enclave of the programme itself.

The limitation of choices in the UK may be the consequence of a much higher degree of standardisation for services provided within the NHS. In the US each level of government (i.e. federal, State, county or municipal) typically sponsors a range of mental health services. In addition, there are many insurance plans, each with its own payment rules. These different payment arrangements, however, rarely impose a strict standard of care. Furthermore, although there is a movement to increase standardisation and quality by implementing evidence-based services in the US (Drake & Goldman, 2003), there is no centralised mechanism for stimulating and guiding this process – nor for monitoring or enforcing such standards. The work of groups like the Cochrane Collaboration, influential in the UK, do not yet have much clout in the US, where the evidence-based practice movement is de-centralised, market-driven, and voluntary (Lehman *et al.*, 2004). Although the variety and choice may be greater in the US, there are specific treatments and services that are in common use in the UK that are almost non-existent in the US. These include cognitive behavioural therapy for enduring mental health problems, early psychosis treatment programmes, and the use of community psychiatric nurses in primary care.

There is more services research and development in the US

Compared to the UK, there is considerably more research and development in mental health services in the US. I am not aware of any study data on the actual figures for such support, but there are many more centres for research and development in America with far more financial support. That difference could also account for the greater variety of services and service innovation in the US. Unfortunately for advocates of evidence-based practice, that innovation is not necessarily followed by widespread adoption of the services that are found to be effective in research and development units.

Federal and State governments sponsor this work in services research and development through several agencies – including National Health Institutes and the Substance Misuse and Mental Health Services Administration – and private foundations – including the MacArthur Foundation and the John A. Hartford Foundation. These activities have launched innovative services over the past several decades, including assertive community treatment (latterly brought to the UK as assertive outreach), integrated treatment for co-occurring substance abuse and mental disorders, supported employment, multi-systemic therapy for children with conduct disorder, and collaborative treatment for depression in primary care settings. They continue to sponsor research and service demonstrations to implement and test various newer services such as 'systems of care' services for children, supported housing, services operated by service users, trauma services and other treatment for post-traumatic stress, and jail diversion programmes.

Over the past several decades the same activities in the UK have been led by a smaller set of centres, such as the Sainsbury Centre for Mental Health, a few research units in medical schools, and more recently by the National Institute for Mental Health in England.

Fragmentation involves different service and policy structures

Poor co-ordination and fragmentation among mental health, general health and social welfare agencies characterise both the US and the UK, but in each country the dysfunctional relationships involve different organisations and structures (DHHS, 2003; DH, 1998a, 1998b). While the NHS is now less centralised than previously, there are many more auspices and sponsors of services in the US, where voluntary organisations and private providers are more numerous than government-operated services. This makes for more opportunities for fragmentation in the US. In the UK there is a complicated and politically sensitive relationship between the NHS and local authorities that is also dysfunctional.

As a result of these structural divisions and historical relationships, both countries experience poor co-ordination of mental health-related services at the local level, particularly between health and social services. In the US, over the past several decades, local mental health authorities have been created to take responsibility for bridging the boundaries. Local mental health authorities provide centralised clinical, administrative, and fiscal responsibility for all citizens who experience a severe mental disorder in a growing number of cities and counties in the US (Shore & Cohen, 1994). In the mid-1990s, SCMH provided a home for several investigators to examine the challenge of local service co-ordination in the UK. They discovered that approaches like joint provision and joint commissioning are favoured over more structural approaches to co-ordination and integration of services, such as local mental health authorities (Hadley & Goldman, 1995, 1998; Shepherd et al., 1996). They concluded, however, that it was critical to co-ordinate the efforts of health and social services and to develop a single point of responsibility for mental health care at the local level.

A new vision of stewardship

Occasioned by this major concern about fragmentation, a new focus on mental health stewardship is emerging in both countries (DHHS, 2003; DH, 1998a, 1998b). The view for the future ought to be on how to meet the complex needs of individuals with mental health problems, particularly those with enduring problems. The challenge for stewardship in the future is to co-ordinate the care of individuals who experience a mental health problem among the diverse agencies that now have some responsibility for this important health and social issue.

The newest catchphrase in mental health policy in the US is 'transformation', connoting the intent to go beyond simple reform to provide a new vision of stewardship for mental health services (DHHS, 2003). It will take more than vision to transform the system, but re-thinking stewardship seems like a sensible place to start. And it is always a good idea to have a vision of where you are going before beginning a journey of epic proportion. Stewardship has also been identified as a key issue for mental health policy worldwide, as reflected in the *World Health Report* (WHO, 2001), and in the UK *National Service Framework for Mental Health* (DH, 1999). Transformation will mean pulling together the efforts of all the agencies that share some degree of responsibility for supporting individuals with mental health problems and aligning policies and financial incentives to make better integrated care possible.

Within health services, transformation will mean better working relationships between inpatient and community services, between primary care and specialist mental health services, and between substance misuse and general psychiatric services. It will also mean more continuity of care among diverse providers in statutory and voluntary sectors. Among the other human service agencies and departments, transformation will mean co-ordination of policy and practice: for children this includes education, child welfare and juvenile justice agencies; for adults it includes employment services, the criminal justice system, and housing authorities.

In a 'transformed' mental health system, fragmentation will be reduced and resources will be used more efficiently because mental health policy will be on the agenda of a wide range of mainstream health and human services agencies. It may be necessary to elevate an individual to the highest levels of government to represent public mental health interests beyond the traditional boundaries of a health service. For example, in the US this might mean appointing a mental health 'czar' within the White House or the Office of the Governor in each of the States. In the UK it might mean appointing someone to carry a mental health portfolio within the Home Office. A renewed focus on mental health at a broad social level would result in policies that affect a wider range of social institutions. It would also result in care plans for individuals and families that promote recovery and reduce the gaps between the potential of new treatments born of scientific advances and the realities of practice with limited resources.

I see this transformation beginning on both sides of the Atlantic. It requires a new vision of stewardship to achieve its promised goals of improved mental health for all our people. Transformation will take ingenuity, resources, and committed organisations like the Sainsbury Centre for Mental Health to achieve the promise.

Acknowledgements

I would like to thank Susan Azrin, PhD, Westat, Inc., and Richard Beinecke, DPA, Suffolk (Massachusetts) University – for their comments and suggestions.

12 Afterword
— From services to human rights

Angela Greatley

Introduction

This book marks a period of 20 or so years of great change in mental health services in the UK. It traces the slow but inexorable move from large old style psychiatric hospitals to more locally-based care. The community-based services that were part of that new pattern of care have themselves grown and developed in that time. Some teams have proved their worth. Others have had to change and new forms of team have been established to augment or replace them, with continuing debate about how to organise care to bring about real improvement for service users. General practitioner services and primary care are also now recognised as a key locus for mental health care, although change here has been slower.

The systems by which local and health authorities plan, provide and commission services have progressed at an ever increasing rate. While commissioning remains underdeveloped, the NHS and local government at least now have a common aim to commission flexible, seamless services and local authorities are beginning to engage with the task of serving their residents who have mental health needs.

Policy links between health and social care have been strengthened, although fragmentation is still evident in practice. More recently a broader range of public policies have been harnessed to address the life experiences of people with mental health problems, for example improving opportunities for real work. The current high profile of public health also affords an opportunity to raise wider concerns about public mental health and well being. However, the experiences of many very disadvantaged people are still unacceptable and will not be tackled until government and mental health services acknowledge the link between mental health and social inequalities.

Perhaps the most significant of all the changes has been that service users and survivors of the mental health system have become commentators on, and increasingly, drivers for change in mental health. Gradually their voices are shifting the mental health world, but not yet the wider public, towards a new way of looking at the lives and the rights of people who experience mental health problems.

Professions are also changing. They have experienced, and sometimes welcomed, increasing challenges to their authority. Roles and responsibilities are now being developed to match the new work. There is also welcome and growing attention to supporting people who have experienced mental health systems to become part of that workforce.

The 20 year period covered by this book almost matches the life span of current mental health legislation. For England and Wales, by the late 1990s the 1983 Act was due for change, based as it was to some degree in the thinking of the late 1950s and rooted in the old institutional care model. It also pre-dated the incorporation of human rights legislation into UK law. In 1998 the mental health world embarked with high hopes on the process that was to lead to a new legislative framework. However, the last seven years have been characterised by growing disappointment with and dismay at the actual proposals made. At the time we publish, we still do not have a legislative framework for England and Wales that will receive broad support. Many now look at the 1983 Act with greater appreciation of the framework it provides. We look forward to learning from Scotland where a different and equally challenging approach has been taken with the new Scottish Mental Health Act.

Other changes to the law, however, are providing new opportunities. It is positive that human rights legislation is on the statute book. It is also positive that people with mental health problems can use the legal framework for disability rights to tackle some of the problems of discrimination from the same perspective as any citizen.

For mental health, this period of change has sometimes been led and always been supported by the Sainsbury Centre for Mental Health (SCMH). Initially formed as the National Unit for Research and Development in Psychiatry in 1985, SCMH, as it is now, has helped to pioneer a new approach to research and evaluation; employing an approach that is action based, front line and relatively rapid.

SCMH has also led work on examining professional roles and on how to ensure the supply of staff to do the job required, as well as how best to prepare and train the existing and future workforce for modern professional practice. It has influenced the development of mental health policy, especially the *National Service Framework for Mental Health* (DH, 1999) through its writing, its conferences and its lobbying. It has worked alongside mental health professionals to develop innovative services and seen these ideas enter the policy framework. Moreover, and perhaps most importantly, SCMH has been part of a support mechanism that has allowed service users to gain a more confident voice and to develop ways of influencing actual service provision.

These next few pages draw out some reflections on what has been and what might be in mental health care, and is written with a mixture of hope, expectation and concern.

How have things changed?

Service users challenging the system

Our 20 year span covers the period when the voice of the people who have used mental health services has emerged and has increased in volume. Both Pilgrim and Campbell offer their perspectives by summarising the history of the service user movement and how individuals and groups have challenged the system. The story includes people labelled as mental patients who stood up and wanted to have their say, people identifying themselves as survivors of the system, as service users, as consumers and as experts by experience. Whatever the position taken and the language that people with mental health problems have chosen to use to describe themselves and their experiences, they have increasingly challenged society's view of what it is to be called mentally ill.

Pilgrim identifies two principal strands in the movement in the UK. Firstly, he identifies the activist, employing the "discourse of activism" where the voice of protest "has been asserted". This often leads people to eschew services and to seek to manage their own approaches to dealing with their experience. The second strand is the growth of service user involvement. The mental health system places value on the reported experience of those who have used services and views are "elicited" with the goal of improving what is offered. Pilgrim also notes, almost in passing, that the views of those who use primary care mental health are hardly audible and that we still fail to distinguish the clear differences of views between service users and those in the carers' movement.

However, Pilgrim challenges user involvement by asking whether people who are coerced into treatment can ever be consumers in service terms and whether consumers can ever challenge the orthodoxies of the psychiatric system. This is an often uncomfortable but ultimately healthy tension. The movement today encompasses individuals and groups occupying different places in this spectrum but also recognises that individuals will take different stances at varying points in their own personal journeys. In order to achieve user-centred care, services have to find ways of acknowledging and valuing the many strands that make up the rich colours and textures of the service user movement. A values-based approach offers real hope for working effectively with different views (Woodbridge & Fulford, 2004).

Campbell reminds us of the achievements of the service user movement. He also recounts how the very act of organising and articulating views has helped individuals to gain greater strength and to challenge myths about the perceived disabilities of people labelled as mentally ill. Wallcraft found almost 900 user groups (Wallcraft et al., 2003). Groups have been taking forward a range of programmes from helping individuals to comment on their own care packages to leadership at the most senior levels in mental health policy and provision. For many this is not without personal cost incurred by challenging the system and by "coming out". As yet, there has been limited support for dealing with these issues from outside the user movement itself. There has been insufficient recognition of the 'burn out' that happens when service users are doing some of the hardest tasks in mental health care with the least resources.

Campbell points out that the biggest challenges arise from the powerlessness engendered by the mental illness label. It keeps people living in poverty; it prevents challenge to the discrimination that is still rife. Even the mental health systems designed to put users at the centre are "honoured only in the breach".

More recently, the proposals for a new Mental Health Act have been a spur for many to pursue the activist road and to challenge the power of compulsion. It may be that this renewed energy will also help in the broader struggle for citizenship. It remains for the mental health community at large to find ways of supporting individuals and groups to articulate their views and to change the system.

Tackling ill health and inequalities

The last few years have seen a welcome interest in public mental health. Gale and Grove remind us that there has been much criticism of the way that mental health has been largely ignored in the broader public health debate. However, it is now an under-pinning theme for public health policy in the UK and it is vital to take this opportunity to drive home the importance of promoting mental health and well being. The most recent statement from the World Health Organization "that there is no health without mental health" (WHO, 2005) sums this up well. We need to press this home in the UK.

There is a growing recognition that social inequalities are a matter for real concern in mental health. The effects of inequalities are seen when access to care is affected by gender, race and class. Power relationships within services can exacerbate these problems and may provide few opportunities for change. Williams and Keating remind us that these issues are often drawn to the attention of the wider society by individuals and groups fighting for civil rights. However, they often remain at the margins of broader policy development.

Mental health staff need to develop an understanding of the way that factors such as poor access, damaging experiences in services and constant challenges to identity affect the most disadvantaged. Services can add to the damage, as the litany of reports into poor treatment of African and Caribbean people shows. Change in the mainstream requires commissioners and staff to challenge social inequalities and begin to improve care for the most disadvantaged.

Services: new for old

Boardman, in his chapter, charts the development of mental health policy in the twentieth century. He reminds us of the relatively short period in which the move from the long stay asylums to locally-based services has really taken root. It seemed grindingly slow as the change was made. But now, two decades on, local community-based services are seen as the core of specialist mental health care.

We applaud these closures for being the first steps on the way to creating the kind of mental health services that service users might well want to see. By closing the institutions society recognised the need to deal with the most distressing examples of abuse and neglect that were found in some of the old hospitals. However, Boardman also reminds us that attention to control remains a central feature of national policy and that this may yet challenge community-based care.

Institutional care does not disappear easily and new forms have come into being. The old hospitals themselves gave birth to some hostels and group homes that have remained institutional in character and inflexible in use. These do not easily help people who have long term mental health problems to have an ordinary life as a tenant of a home of their own.

The 1990s saw rising rates of detention under the Mental Health Act. While this seems to have levelled off, rates remain very high. There is some evidence, as Warner reminds us, that new forms of secure care have grown and, indeed, have been said to have consumed some of the early growth in the new investment for mental health services in the late 1990s.

Whatever the pattern of service it has to be of good quality and provide decent standards. Warner reminds us of the troubled history of inpatient hospital care. In many places accommodation still remains unfit for a modern mental health service. Staffing provides a considerable challenge. The range and availability of therapies is very variable and many inpatients report boredom and lack of care. Government has to deal with the worst accommodation and with poor therapeutic input as a matter of urgency and certainly before the end of the ten-year implementation period for the *National Service Framework*.

As we move into the era where community-based services are the norm there is no shortage of debate about the form it should take. Onyett takes us to the heart of the current discussions: how best to re-engineer the system to put the service user at its heart.

In the first five years of the *NSF* we have seen new teams emerge. Some have a clear sense of purpose and an understanding of the meaning of their work as they break new ground, while others struggle to tick boxes. However, the "hostility" that can be seen between teams is not new. It echoes the changes of 20 years ago and the end-stage of the closure of the large psychiatric hospitals. Then, the 'new kids on the block', the community mental health centres, were drawing staff from the old hospitals and changing the centre of gravity in mental health care. It became clear then that the only way forward was for the service to understand the relationships with others and how a system had to be created to serve the patients – a lesson that was learned but not always acted upon. In the current situation, this means looking at the whole system, offering clear leadership and focusing on what is known to work if the new teams are going to be able to deliver high quality care.

Primary mental health care remains an area in need of increased attention. Cohen outlines the changing face of general practice and the growth of a more broadly based primary care service. He charts how successive governments have seen primary care as a key component in shifting the whole way in which the NHS functions. With a place in the *National Service Framework for Mental Health* and the growing wealth of guidelines from the National Institute for Clinical Excellence and other bodies, the place of primary care at the heart of mental care is assured, but delivery is slow.

Despite significant changes it is not surprising that all of our contributors share the view that a great deal remains on the 'to do' list for mental health care in the UK. There seems to be some degree of willingness to tackle these issues at present, but significant change requires a paradigm shift in thinking about services and about the funding needed.

Resources for mental health care

Parsonage's chapter reminds us that there is much to be done to ensure equity of access in mental health care. The distribution of newer style services is patchy and there are still significant gaps in provision. There is considerable concern about the distribution of resources between different groups and different forms of provision and a postcode lottery of unexplained difference persists.

It is often difficult to be clear about the extent of these differences because information on spending in mental health remains hard to obtain. What can be seen is a major increase in spending by health and local government on mental health services over the last 20 years, plus a shift in that spending from inpatient to community services. There are still concerns, however, that growth in funding for mental health and social care has increased at a slower rate than NHS and social care overall. Mental health care still needs more funding but also needs to tackle inefficiencies. Investment in better information is now critical and mental health care risks falling back if this does not happen.

A key priority is to strengthen commissioning. Commissioners need to take more responsibility for ensuring that services are appropriate and that they join up as public services move to a more mixed economy of care. The growth of provision by the voluntary sector, where flexibility and responsiveness may be easier to achieve, has been widely welcomed. Many, though not all, also recognise the important contribution of the private sector, sometimes in specialist areas. It is widely recognised that diversity in service provision is more likely to offer solutions that are responsive to individuals.

All of this progress may yet be halted by problems in getting the right staff into the right places at the right time. In the late eighties it is clear that insufficient attention was paid to the need to plan for and nurture mental health staff. There have been significant changes since that time. Staff groups that were novel in the last half of the twentieth century, like community mental health nurses, have become a bedrock of care and are being joined by very new groups like primary care mental health workers. Professions are changing their roles and responsibilities in an effort to match the needs of the new style services.

Philip reminds us of the great strides being made at national and regional level to recruit, retain, train and develop a modern mental health workforce. Yet he questions whether this will be sufficient to deal with the scale of the problem. Philip suggests that more radical action will be required including new patterns for service delivery employing a greater diversity of providers as well as tapping into newer labour markets.

All of these pressures require commissioners and providers to work closely together. Yet fragmentation is still evident in arrangements for planning, commissioning and providing mental health services. Goldman reminds us that, unlike some other countries, the UK still benefits from an entitlement to health care free at the point of delivery, of the responsibilities of local government in social welfare and of duties to work together. Yet the experience of service users remains one of poor co-ordination and disjointed services. Whatever the particular configuration of commissioning agencies, they have to take responsibility for developing a framework for services that is built on an understanding of the patterns of care that individuals want.

What about the next twenty years?

A new focus

In his foreword to this book, Matt Muijen draws our attention to the "tremendous transformation" that has taken place over the last 20 years of mental health care. What do we want to see in the next 20 and what might we expect? What is clear is that the focus of concern and action needs to move away from services towards a valued life in society. We need to achieve a better balance between promoting good mental health, supporting and treating people with mental health problems and working for social inclusion.

For this to happen, mental health and well being need to become more fully integrated into the mainstream agenda for public health. This requires a greater understanding of the determinants of good mental health plus action to counter the adverse social, economic and political factors that contribute to poor mental health. Mental health and well being are rarely a matter for individual lifestyle choice and are closely connected with social and family environments. Measures to tackle these problems both promote well being and offer supportive environments to those who do develop mental health problems. This is a big agenda for the next 20 years.

Discrimination and stigma have to be challenged head-on. We have seen how discrimination leads to unjust treatment and exclusion of people with mental health problems and particularly of those with serious and long term difficulties. The negative stereotypes carried by the national media alone show how the life chances of people with mental health problems are damaged by the views of others. There is a growing, though as yet incomplete, understanding of what works in countering discrimination and this provides an agenda for the next quarter century and beyond. This is often said to be very difficult work and it has proved to be so in the past.

But there are some ways in which we can begin tackling the problem. Public authorities need to provide the support that will enable individuals and groups of people with mental health problems to live and work in the community. Meeting and talking with others in society is a powerful way of breaking down barriers. Information and education is needed for public and private organisations to counter negative stereotypes. This should include challenging the media if they perpetuate these stereotypes.

Some people with mental health problems will use the legal frameworks of human rights and anti-discrimination to push the barriers away; again support will be needed to make this possible. By whatever means people with mental health problems choose to tackle the issues, society has to take responsibility for challenging discrimination.

Securing employment, housing, access to services and participation in community life for people with mental health problems will be key goals for the next 20 years. Much is known about the effects of low income and multiple disadvantages on people with mental health problems. There is some evidence of a willingness to tackle these issues nationally and locally, but this is a matter for sustained effort and progress will probably be very slow.

Special attention will be needed to counter social inequalities. There is now recognition of the problems faced by people from Black and minority ethnic communities, by women and by people who become caught up in the criminal justice system and experience very poor mental health care. Tackling these failings must be seen as core business for every-one working in mental health care, not a side issue away from mainstream activity.

All of the above form a formidable agenda for action and will require sustained pressure from national and local authorities and all mental health stakeholders to achieve good outcomes. However, shifts in attitude and public policy rarely achieve smooth and sus-tained forward progress. There are many negative aspects to the current environment that may prove to be considerable barriers to progress. Attitudes to risk and dangerousness may be leading professionals to err on the side of extreme caution and can contribute to society's fear of people with mental health problems.

The proposed mental health legislation is seen by many as a considerable challenge. The right kind of legislation, based on rights and respecting an individual's capacity to make decisions, is vital. Achieving this is no easy task – we still face a hostile political climate where fears about violence take precedence over concerns for the human rights of individuals with severe mental health problems. Yet without a genuinely modern legal framework that attains the right balance, efforts to tackle stigma and make services more responsive to users will be seriously compromised.

Changing services

The debate about care and control swirls around mental health services at the start of this century as it did throughout the last, and even earlier than that. Mental health and primary care services should be about helping people who experience problems to meet their needs for support and treatment, offering a range of responses and helping them to achieve their aspirations: as Gale and Grove put it "Supporting people to undertake their personal journey to a better life...". Some people will want to use medication, very many want access to talking therapies, and all want services that are respectful and responsive. Practice has to change radically and will involve professionals giving up some of their power and striking new relationships with the people who use services.

For some service users this discussion is framed in terms of recovery. Recovery is described as a process of growing and overcoming challenges that is unique and personal. It has made an impact on national policy and, in some other countries, has led to a new way of designing services. It offers an opportunity for the two key strands of the service user movement to come together in the quest for responsive and respectful services that enable individuals to get the support they want to live the lives that they determine. The debate is still at an early stage in the UK but must have a major influence on the ways that services change in the years to come. Recovery is seen as personally empowering and has been said to offer a "realistic hope for a better life alongside whatever remains of illness" (Roberts & Wolfson, 2004).

Choice has also come on to the Government's agenda for the NHS. To date, mental health has not been much included, but the debate could offer a further opportunity to drive change in services. The debate to date has centred on possible 'distortions' in the health care system. There has been polarisation between positions that might be characterised as 'all people need is good services' and 'choice will drive the system to provide better solutions'. However, a more subtle discussion about choice and responsiveness has something to offer for mental health.

Firstly, service user views are needed at the point of design and re-design of services. There is an opportunity to re-iterate the call for a broader range of services, including talking therapies. Secondly, people need clear and accessible information if they are to make choices, and information is one of the things that service users have wanted over the last 20 years. Access is a central aspect of responsive services. In mental health many people ask for support but are turned away and do not get help until they become very distressed; the last 20 years has sadly demonstrated how this affects people from African and Caribbean communities, amongst many. Few of us would expect to be denied health care when we ask for it only to be forced to accept what we do not want, possibly under compulsion, at a later stage. The debate about choice and responsiveness should not be ignored and could be another driver for change in mental health services.

The *National Service Framework* has been a huge step forward for mental health care in the UK and much has been achieved, though work remains to be completed. For the short to medium term it provides the targets to be achieved if we are to finish the job that started with the closure of the water tower hospitals. The National Director for Mental Health provided a clear account of the work agenda in his five year review (DH, 2004).

All of the areas discussed deserve investment and action and it is seems invidious to select any one for special attention. But there is one area of mental health care that is in desperate need of improvement. Acute inpatient care is the most pressing piece of unfinished NHS business in the short term. The list of problems remains considerable in too many inpatient units: the environment, the patient's day, staffing, therapies, activities, care planning, designing care to support inclusion, dealing with disturbance and co-existing substance misuse are just some of the items in need of urgent attention. We hope to see a real change in the near future.

For the Sainsbury Centre for Mental Health, the challenge will be to play a continuing part in shaping the agenda while also supporting implementation and monitoring progress towards it. As we enter our third decade in operation, SCMH will have a clear focus on some of the most critical areas of concern: of getting the right workforce for the future; of improving systems of care; of making recovery and social inclusion a reality for service users; and of ensuring services respond better to the needs of the most excluded and poorly served people.

This is a massive undertaking at the best of times. While much of it is supported by the current policy environment, the political climate is always subject to change and in some ways remains hostile. As this book shows, mental health services are often at the mercy of trends in policy and politics over which they have little or no influence.

So if there is one further challenge for all of us who are concerned about mental health, from whichever standpoint, it is to work as far as we can to help to shape the political landscape: to take mental health from the margins of public policy to the centre and to make the needs and wishes of people with mental health problems heard by those with the power to make a difference to them.

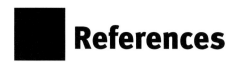

References

Chapter 1: Protest and Co-Option – The voice of mental health service users

Barham, P. & Hayward, R. (1991) *From the Mental Patient to the Person*. London: Routledge.

Barnes, M. & Shardlow, P. (1997) From passive recipient to active citizen: participation in mental health user groups. *Journal of Mental Health*, **6**, 289-300.

Baruch, G. & Treacher, A. (1977) *Psychiatry Observed*. London: RKP.

Beresford, P. & Croft, S. (1986) *Whose Welfare? Private Care or Public Service*. London: Lewis Cohen Urban Studies.

Bhui, K., Aubin, A. & Strathdee, G. (1998) Making a reality of user involvement in community mental health services. *Psychiatric Bulletin*, **22**, 8-11.

Bowl, R. (1996) Involving service users in mental health services: social services departments and the NHS and Community Care Act 1990. *Journal of Mental Health*, **5** (3) 287-303.

Burstow, B. & Weitz, D. (eds) (1988) *Shrink Resistant: The Struggle Against Psychiatry in Canada*. Vancouver: New Star.

Campbell, P. (1996) The history of the user movement in the United Kingdom. In: Heller, T., Reynolds, J., Gomm, R., Murston, R. & Pattison, S. (eds) *Mental Health Matters*. Basingstoke: Macmillan.

Campbell, J. & Schraiber, R. (1989) *In Pursuit of Wellness: The Well-Being Project*. Sacramento: Californian Department of Health.

Carter, M.F. (2003) The relationship of a self-reported assessment of need in mental illness to insight. *Journal of Mental Health*, **12** (1) 81-90.

Chamberlin, J. (1977) *On Our Own*. London: Mind.

Crossley, M.L. & Crossley, N. (2001) 'Patient' voices, social movements and the habitus: how psychiatric survivors 'speak out'. *Social Science and Medicine*, **52** (10) 1477-1489.

Diamond, B., Parkin, G., Morris, K., Bettinis, J. & Bettesworth, C. (2003) User involvement: substance or spin? *Journal of Mental Health*, **12** (6) 613-626.

Guze, S. (1989) Biological psychiatry: is there any other kind? *Psychological Medicine*, **19**, 315-323.

Haafkens, J., Nijhof, G. & van der Poel, E. (1986) Mental health care and the opposition movement in the Netherlands. *Social Science and Medicine*, **22**, 185-92.

Habermas, J. (1981) New social movements. *Telos*, **48**, 33-7.

Hatfield, B., Huxley, P. & Hadi, M. (1992) Accommodation and employment: a survey into the circumstances and expressed needs of the users of mental health services in a northern town. *British Journal of Social Work*, **22** (4) 32–50.

Kay, A. & Legg, C. (1986) *Discharged into the Community*. London: Good Practices in Mental Health.

MacDonald, G. & Sheldon, B. (1997) Community care services for the mentally ill: consumers' views. *International Journal of Social Psychiatry*, **43** (1) 35–55.

Mayer, J. & Timms, N. (1970) *The Client Speaks*. London: Routledge & Kegan Paul.

Mind (2004) *Ward Watch: Mind's campaign to improve hospital conditions for mental health patients*. Available from: http://www.mind.org.uk/News+policy+and+campaigns/ [Accessed 22 February 2005]

Pilgrim, D. & Waldron, L. (1998) User involvement in mental health services: how far can it go? *Journal of Mental Health*, **7** (1) 95-104.

Rogers, A. (1993) Coercion and voluntary admission: an examination of psychiatric patients' views. *Behavioral Sciences and the Law*, **11**, 259-267.

Rogers, A. & Pilgrim, D. (1991) Pulling down churches: accounting for the mental health users' movement. *Sociology of Health and Illness*, **13** (2) 129-48.

Rogers, A. & Pilgrim, D. (2001) Users and their advocates. In: Thornicroft, G. & Szmukler, G. (eds) *Textbook of Community Psychiatry*. Oxford: Oxford University Press.

Rogers, A. & Pilgrim, D. (2003) *Mental Health and Inequality*. Basingstoke: Palgrave.

Rogers, A., Pilgrim, D. & Lacey, R. (1993) *Experiencing Psychiatry: Users' Views of Services*. Basingstoke: Mind/Macmillan.

Romme, M. & Escher, S. (1993) *Accepting Voices*. London: Mind.

Rose, D. (2003) Partnership, co-ordination of care and the place of user involvement. *Journal of Mental Health*, **12** (1) 59-70.

Rutter, D., Manley, C., Weaver T., Crawford, M.J. & Fulop, N. (2004). Patients or partners? Case studies in user involvement in the planning and delivery of adult mental health services in London. *Social Science and Medicine*, **58** (10) 1973-1984.

The Sainsbury Centre for Mental Health (1998) *Acute Problems: A Survey of the Quality of Care in Acute Psychiatric Wards*. London: SCMH.

Sayce, L. (2000) *From Psychiatric Patient to Citizen: Overcoming discrimination and social exclusion*. Basingstoke: Macmillan.

Stone, M. (1985) Shellshock and the psychologists. In: Bynum, W.F., Porter, R. & Shepherd M. (eds) *The Anatomy of Madness*, Vol. 2. London: Tavistock.

Toch, H. (1965) *The Social Psychology of Social Movements*. New York: Bobbs Merrill.

Truman, C. & Raine, P. (2002) Experience and meaning of user involvement: some explorations from a community mental health project. *Health and Social Care in the Community* **10**, (3) 136-143.

Chapter 2: New Services for Old – An overview of mental health policy

Audit Commission (1986) *Making a Reality of Community Care*. London: HMSO.

Audit Commission (1992) *Community Care: Managing the Cascade of Change*. London: HMSO.

Audit Commission (1994) *Finding a Place. A Review of Mental Health Services for Adults*. London: HMSO.

Barratt, Sir C., James, Lady, Jones, R.H. & Lane, W.E. (1968) *Report of the Committee on Local Authority and Allied Personal Social Services*. London: HMSO.

Bateson, G. (1972) *Steps to an Ecology of Mind*. New York: Ballantine Books.

Department of Health (1992) *Health of the Nation White Paper*. London: HMSO.

Department of Health (1999) *National Service Framework for Mental Health: Modern Standards and Service Models*. London: DH.

Department of Health (2000) *The NHS Plan: A plan for investment, a plan for reform*. London: DH.

Department of Health (2001) *The National Service Framework for Older People*. London: DH.

Department of Health (2004a) *The National Service Framework for Mental Health – Five years on*. London: DH.

Department of Health (2004b) *Mental Health Care Group Workforce Team: National Mental Health Workforce Strategy*. London: DH.

Department of Health (2004c) *The National Service Framework for Children, Young People and Maternity Services: The mental health and psychological wellbeing of children and young people*. London: DH.

Department of Health (2005) *Delivering Race Equality in Mental Health Care: An Action Plan for Reform Inside and Outside Services and The Government's Response to the Independent Inquiry into the Death of David Bennett*. London: DH.

Department of Health and Social Security (1969) *Report of the Committee of Inquiry into Allegations of Ill-treatment of patients and other irregularities at the Ely Hospital, Cardiff.* London: HMSO.

Department of Health and Social Security (1971) *Hospital Services for the Mentally Ill.* London: HSMO.

Department of Health and Social Security (1975) *Better Services for the Mentally Ill.* London: HSMO.

Department of Health and Social Security (1985) *Community Care with special reference to adult mentally ill and mentally handicapped people.* London: HMSO.

Department of Health and Social Security (1988) *Report of the Committee of Inquiry into the Care and Aftercare of Miss Sharon Campbell.* London: HMSO.

Griffiths, Sir R. (1984) *NHS Management Enquiry Report. Social Services Committee.* London: HMSO.

Griffiths, Sir R. (1988) *Community Care: Agenda for Action. A Report to the Secretary of State for Social Services by Sir Roy Griffiths.* London: HMSO.

Hall, S. & Jacques, M. (eds) (1983) *The Politics of Thatcherism.* London: Lawrence and Wishart.

Healthcare Commission (2004) *Rating the NHS: NHS Performance Ratings 2003/4.* London: Commission for Health Care Audit and Inspection. Available from: http://www.chi.nhs.uk/eng/ratings/index.shtml [Accessed 7 March 2005]

Hill, D. (1969) *Psychiatry in Medicine. Retrospect and Prospect.* London: Nuffield Provincial Hospitals Trust.

House of Commons (1990) *The National Health Service and Community Care Act.* London: HMSO.

Jones, K. (1972) *A History of the Mental Health Services.* London: Routledge and Kegan Paul.

Laing, R.D. (1960) *The Divided Self.* London: Tavistock.

Laing, R.D. & Esterson, A. (1964) *Sanity, Madness and the Family.* London: Tavistock.

Laugharne, R. (2004) Psychiatry in the Future. The next 15 years: postmodern challenges and opportunities for psychiatry. *Psychiatric Bulletin,* **28,** 317-318.

Ministry of Health (1962) *A Hospital Plan for England and Wales.* London: HMSO.

Ministry of Health (1963) *Health and Welfare: the Development of Community Care.* London: HMSO.

Odegard, O. (1964) Pattern of discharge from Norwegian psychiatric hospitals before and after the introduction of psychotropic drugs. *American Journal of Psychiatry,* **120,** 772-778.

Pollock, A.M. (2004) *NHS plc. The Privatisation of Our Healthcare.* London: Verso.

Ramon, S. (1982) The Logic of Pragmatism in Mental Health Policy: The implications of the government position on mental health in the 1959 debate for the 80s. *Critical Social Policy,* **2,** 38-54.

Ritchie, J., Dick, D. & Lingham, R. (1994) *The Report of the Inquiry into the Care and Treatment of Christopher Clunis.* London: HMSO.

Rollin, H.R. (1977) 'De-institutionalisation' and the community: fact and fiction. *Psychological Medicine,* **7,** 181-184.

Rose, N. (2001) Historical changes in mental health practice. In: Thornicroft, G. & Szmukler, G. (eds) *Textbook of Community Psychiatry.* Oxford: Oxford University Press.

Rosenhan, D.I. (1973) On being sane in insane places. *Science,* **179,** 250-258.

The Sainsbury Centre for Mental Health (2003) *Money for Mental Health: A review of public spending on mental health care.* London: SCMH.

Sayce, E., Craig, T.K.J. & Boardman, A.P. (1991) Community Mental Health Centres in the United Kingdom. *Social Psychiatry Psychiatric Epidemiology,* **26,** 14-20.

Shepherd, M., Goodman, S. & Watt, D.C. (1961) The application of Hospital Statistics in the evaluation of pharmacotherapy in a psychiatric population. *Comprehensive Psychiatry,* **2,** 1-9.

Social Exclusioin Unit (2004) *Mental Health and Social Exclusion. Social Exclusion Unit Report.* London: ODPM.

Szasz, T.S. (1961) *The Myth of Mental illness*. London: Secker and Warburg.

Titmuss, R. (1961) Community Care, fact or fiction? (Annual conference Report, National Association for Mental Health). Reprinted in: Freeman, H. & Farndale, J. (eds) (1963) *Trends in mental health services*. London: Pergammon.

Wilkinson, R. G. (1996) *Unhealthy Societies. The Afflictions of Inequality*. London: Routledge.

Wing, J.K. & Brown, G.W. (1970) *Institutionalism and Schizophrenia: A comparative study of three mental hospitals 1960-1968*. Cambridge: Cambridge University Press.

Chapter 3: Acute Care in Crisis

Antoniou. J. (2000) Back in one piece. *Nursing Times,* **96** (40) 23-24.

Audit Commission (1986) *Making a Reality of Community Care*. London: HMSO.

Barker, D. (2000) *Environmentally Friendly? Patients' views of conditions on psychiatric wards.* London: Mind.

Blom-Cooper, L., Hally, H. & Murphy, E. (1995) *The Falling Shadow – one patient's mental health care 1978-1993.* London: Duckworth.

Clarke, S. (2004) *Acute Inpatient Mental Health Care: Education, Training and Professional Development for All.* London: The National Institute for Mental Health in England/The Sainsbury Centre for Mental Health.

Colgan, S. (2002) Who wants to be a general psychiatrist? *Psychiatric Bulletin,* **26**, 3-4.

Commission for Health Improvement (2003) *What CHI has found in mental health trusts. Sector report*. London: Commission for Health Improvement.

Department of Health (1993) *Health of the Nation Key Area Handbook: Mental Illness*. London: DH.

Department of Health (1996) *The spectrum of care: local services for people with mental health problems*. Wetherby: DH.

Department of Health (1997) *The New NHS: Modern, Dependable*. London: DH.

Department of Health (1998a) *A First Class Service: Quality in the New NHS*. London: DH.

Department of Health (1998b) *Modernising Mental Health Services: Safe, Sound and Supportive*. London: DH.

Department of Health (1999) *National Service Framework for Mental Health: Modern Standards and Service Models*. London: DH.

Department of Health (2000) *The NHS Plan: A plan for investment, a plan for reform*. London: DH.

Department of Health (2001) *The Mental Health Policy Implementation Guide*. London: DH.

Department of Health (2002) *Mental Health Policy Implementation Guide – Adult Acute Inpatient Care Provision*. London: DH.

Department of Health (2004a) *DoH Form KH03. Average daily number of available beds, by sector, England, 1987-88 to 2003-04.* Available from: http://www.performance.doh.gov. uk/hospitalactivity/ [Accessed 2 March 2005]

Department of Health (2004b) *Form KH03. Hospital Inpatient Activity: Average daily number of available and occupied beds by ward classification, England, 2003-04.* Available from: http://www.performance.doh. gov.uk/hospitalactivity/ [Accessed 2 March 2005]

Department of Health (2004c) *Statistical Bulletin. In-patients formally detained in hospitals under the Mental Health Act 1983 and other legislation, England: 1993-94 to 2003-04.* Bulletin 2004/22. Available from: http://www.publications.doh.gov.uk/public/ sb0422.htm [Accessed 22 February 2005]

Department of Health and Social Security (1975) *Better Services for the Mentally Ill.* London: HMSO.

Department of Health and Social Security (1989) *Caring for People: Community Care in the Next Decade and Beyond*. London: HMSO.

Griffiths, Sir R. (1988) *Community Care: Agenda for Action. A Report to the Secretary of State for Social Services by Sir Roy Griffiths*. London: HMSO.

Health Service Journal (2004) *Fit for purpose.* Available from: http://www.hsj.co.uk/nav?page=hsj.mentalhealth [Accessed 22 February 2005]

Hoult. J., Reynolds, I., Charbonneau-Powis, M., Weekes, P. & Briggs, J. (1983) Psychiatric hospital versus community treatment: the results of a randomised trial. *Australian and New Zealand Journal of Psychiatry,* **17**, 160-167.

House of Commons (1990) *The National Health Service and Community Care Act.* London: HMSO

Johnson, S. & Thornicroft, G. (1991) Emergency psychiatric services in England and Wales. In: Phelan, M., Strathdee, G. & Thornicroft, G. (eds) *Emergency Mental Health Services.* Cambridge: Cambridge University Press.

Kennedy, P. & Griffiths, H. (2001) General psychiatrists discovering new roles for a new era ... and removing work stress. *British Journal of Psychiatry,* **179** (4) 283-285.

Laurance, J. (2002) *Pure madness: how fear drives the mental health system.* London: King's Fund/Faculty of Public Health Medicine.

Lawson, B. & Phiri, M. (1999) *The architectural healthcare environment and its effect on patient health outcomes.* Sheffield: University of Sheffield.

Lawson, B. & Phiri, M. (2000) Room for improvement. *Health Service Journal,* **110** (5688) 24-27.

Mahoney, J. (2004) *Outcome of Hospital Closure Programme.* London: National Institute for Mental Health in England. Available from: http://www.fic.nih.gov/dcpp/ppts/mahoney.ppt [Accessed 2 March 2005]

McGeorge, M. & Lindow, V. (2000) Safe in our hands? *Mental Health Practice,* **4** (4) 4-5.

Mental Health Act Commission (2004) *Count Me In: National Mental Health and Ethnicity Census 2005 (England and Wales).* Available from: http://www.mhac.org.uk/census/ [Accessed 22 February 2005]

Mental Health Foundation/The Sainsbury Centre for Mental Health (2002) *Being There in a Crisis: A report of the learning from eight mental health crisis services.* London: Mental Health Foundation.

Mind (1999) *Creating Accepting Communities – Social Exclusion and Mental Health Problems, Report of Mind Inquiry.* London: Mind.

Mind (2004) *Ward Watch: Mind's campaign to improve hospital conditions for mental health patients.* Available from: http://www.mind.org.uk/News+policy+and+campaigns/ [Accessed 22 February 2005]

Minghella, E., Ford, R., Freeman, T., Hoult, J., McGlynn, P. & O'Halloran, P. (1998) *Open All Hours: 24-hour response for people with mental health emergencies.* London: The Sainsbury Centre for Mental Health.

Muijen, M. (2002) Acute wards: problems and solutions. *Psychiatric Bulletin,* **26**, 342-343.

National Institute for Mental Health in England (2003) *Cases for Change. Policy Context.* London: NIMHE.

The National Institute for Mental Health in England/Changing Workforce Provision/The Royal College of Psychiatrists/Department of Health (2004) *Guidance on new ways of working for psychiatrists in a multi-disciplinary and multi-agency context: National Steering Group interim report.* London: DH.

National Institute for Mental Health in England (2004) *The Ten Essential Shared Capabilities – A framework for the whole of the mental health workforce.* London: DH.

The National Health Service Executive (2000) *Safety, Privacy and Dignity in Mental Health Units. Guidance on mixed sex accommodation for mental health units.* London: DH.

Orme, S. & Hogan, K. (2000) *Crisis Services in the UK – Report of a nation-wide survey of UK crisis services.* Wolverhampton: University of Wolverhampton.

Powell, E. (1961) Available from: http://www.mdx.ac.uk/www/study/xpowell.htm [Accessed 26.01.05]

Priebe, S., Badesconyi, A., Fioritti, A., Hansson, H., Kilian, R., Torres-Gonzales, F., Turner, T. & Wiersma, D. (2005) Reinstitutionalisation in mental health care: comparison of data on service provision from six European countries. *British Medical Journal,* **330**, 123-126.

Rose, D. (2001) *Users' Voices: The perspectives of mental health service users on community and hospital care.* London: The Sainsbury Centre for Mental Health.

Royal College of Psychiatrists (1998) *Not just bricks and mortar. Council report CR62.* London: Royal College of Psychiatrists.

The Sainsbury Centre for Mental Health and Mental Health Act Commission (1997) *The National Visit: A one-day Visit to 309 Acute Psychiatric Wards by the Mental Health Act Commission in collaboration with the Sainsbury Centre for Mental Health.* London: SCMH.

The Sainsbury Centre for Mental Health (1998) *Acute Problems: A survey of the quality of care in acute psychiatric wards.* London: SCMH.

The Sainsbury Centre for Mental Health (2001) *The Capable Practitioner: A framework and list of the practitioner capabilities required to implement the National Service Framework for Mental Health.* Available from: http://www.scmh.org.uk/8025695100388752/vWeb/wpASTN4XLCX8?opendocument [Accessed 22 February 2005]

The Sainsbury Centre for Mental Health (2002) *The Search for Acute Solutions.* Available from: http://www.scmh.org.uk/8025694D00337EF1/vWeb/fsCPIR4PDJ8Q [Accessed 26 January 2005]

Stein, L. & Test, M. (1980) An alternative to mental hospital treatment. *Archives of General Psychiatry,* **37**, 392-299.

Stewart, G. (2003) *Key dates in the history of mental health and community care.* Available from: http://www.mind.org.uk/Information/Factsheets/History+of+mental+health/ [Accessed 26 January 2005]

Warner, L., Nicholas, S., Patel, K., Harris, J. & Ford, R. (2000) *National Visit 2: Improving Care for Detained Patients from Black and Minority Ethnic Communities. A visit by the Mental Health Act Commission to 104 Mental Health and Learning Disability Units in England and Wales.* London: The Sainsbury Centre for Mental Health.

Warner, L., Hoadley, A., Braithwaite, T., Barnes, A., Lamb, D. & Lindley, P. (2003) *The Search for Acute Solutions: Preliminary Report.* Unpublished. London: The Sainsbury Centre for Mental Health.

Chapter 4: Mental Health Workforce

Audit Commission (2002) *Recruitment and Retention: A public service workforce for the twenty-first century.* London: Audit Commission.

Bach, S. (1998) NHS Pay determination and work re-organisation, Employee Relations Reform in NHS Trusts. *The International Journal of Employee Relations,* **20** (6) p.565-576.

Barnett, S., Buchanan, D., Patrickson, M. & Maddem, J. (1996) Negotiating the evolution of the HR function: Practical advice from the healthcare sector. *Human Resource Management Journal,* **6** (4) 18-37.

Commission for Health Improvement (2003) *What CHI has found in mental health trusts. Sector report.* London: Commission for Health Improvement.

Department of Health (1998a) *Modernising Social Services: Promoting independence, improving protection, raising standards.* London: DH.

Department of Health (1998b) *Modernising Mental Health Services: Safe, Sound and Supportive.* London: DH.

Department of Health (1998c) *Working Together: Securing a quality workforce for the NHS.* London: DH.

Department of Health (1999) *National Service Framework for Mental Health: Modern Standards and Service Models.* London: DH.

Department of Health (2000a) *The NHS Plan: A plan for investment, a plan for reform.* London: DH.

Department of Health (2000b) *A Health Service of all the talents: Developing the NHS workforce.* London: DH.

Department of Health (2001a) *The Mental Health Policy Implementation Guide.* London: DH.

Department of Health (2001b) *The National Service Framework for Older People.* London: DH.

Department of Health (2002a) *HR in the NHS Plan: More staff working differently.* London: DH.

Department of Health (2002b) *Delivering the NHS Plan: Next steps on investment, next steps on reform.* London: DH.

Department of Health (2004a) *The National Service Framework for Children, Young People and Maternity Services: The mental health and psychological wellbeing of children and young people*. London: DH.

Department of Health (2004b) *The NHS Knowledge and Skills Framework (NHS KSF) and the Development Review Process*. London: DH.

Department of Health (2004c) *NHS Job Evaluation Handbook Second Edition*. London: DH.

Department of Health (2004d) *The National Service Framework for Mental Health – Five years on*. London: DH.

Department of Health (2004e) *Mental Health Care Group Workforce Team: National Mental Health Workforce Strategy*. London: DH.

Farnham, D. & Horton, S. (1996) *Managing the New Public Services*. Basingstoke: MacMillan Press.

Flanagan, H. (1998) Human Resource Management in the NHS – AD 2001. In: Sturgeon, P. (ed) *The New Face of the NHS*. Second edition. London: Royal Society of Medicine Press.

Flynn, N. (2002) *Public Sector Management*. Harlow: Pearson Education Limited.

Genkeer, L., Gough, P. & Finlayson, B. (2003) *London's Mental Health Workforce: A review of recent developments*. London: King's Fund.

Griffiths, R. (1984) *NHS Management Enquiry Report*. Social Services Committee. London: HMSO.

House of Commons Select Committee on Health (1999) *Future NHS staffing requirements*. Third Report. London, HMSO.

Huxley, P., Evans, S., Gately, C. & Webber, M. (2003) *Workload and Working Patterns of Mental Health Social Workers: an investigation into occupational pressures*. London: Institute of Psychiatry.

Mangan, P. (1994) The Collapse of the Conventional Career. *Nursing Times*, **90** (16) 21-31.

Morton-Cooper, A. & Bamford, M. (1997) *Excellence in Healthcare Management*. Oxford: Blackwell Science Ltd.

National Institute for Mental Health in England (2004) *The Ten Essential Shared Capabilities – A framework for the whole of the mental health workforce*. London: DH.

Regional Manpower Planners Group (1988) *The Black Hole*. NHS internal report. Unpublished.

Rogers, A. & Pilgrim, D. (2001) *Mental Health Policy in Britain*. Second edition. Hampshire: Palgrave.

The Sainsbury Centre for Mental Health (1997) *Pulling Together: The future roles and training of mental health staff*. London: SCMH.

The Sainsbury Centre for Mental Health (2000) *Finding and Keeping: Review of recruitment and retention in the mental health workforce*. London, SCMH

The Sainsbury Centre for Mental Health (2001) *The Capable Practitioner: A framework and list of the practitioner capabilities required to implement the National Service Framework for Mental Health*. Available from: http://www.scmh.org.uk/8025695100388752/vWeb/wpASTN4XLCX8?opendocument [Accessed 22 February 2005]

The Sainsbury Centre for Mental Health (2003) *A Mental Health Workforce for the Future: A planners guide*. London: SCMH.

Skills for Health (2003) *Mental Health Standards framework*. Final version. Available from: http://www.skillsforhealth.org.uk/standards_database/index.htm [Accessed 7 March 2005]

Topss England (2000) *Modernising the Social Care Workforce – the first national training strategy for England*. Available from: http://www.topss.org.uk [Accessed 7 March 2005]

Topss England Workforce Intelligence Unit (2003) The State of the Social Care Workforce in England, summary of the first annual report of the Topss England Workforce Intelligence Unit. Available from: http://www.topss.org.uk [Accessed 7 March 2005]

The Workforce Action Team (2001) *Adult Mental Health: National Service Framework (and the NHS Plan) Underpinning Programme: Workforce, Education and Training*. London: DH.

Sources for workforce data

Department of Health (1989) *NHS Workforce in England: Nursing and Midwifery and Professions Allied to Medicine*. London: DH.

Department of Health (1993) *Health and Personal Social Services Statistics for England*. London: DH.

Department of Health (1994) *Health and Personal Social Services Statistics for England*. London: DH.

Department of Health (1995) *NHS Workforce in England*. London: DH.

Department of Health (2003) *Personal Social Services staff of Social Services Departments at 30 September 2003, England*. London: DH.

Department of Health (2004) *The National Service Framework for Mental Health – Five years on*. London: DH.

Chapter 5: The Mental Health Economy

Audit Commission (2003) *Achieving the NHS Plan*. London: Audit Commission Publications.

Aziz, F., McCrone, P., Boyle, S. & Knapp, M. (2003) *Financing Mental Health Services in London: central funding and local expenditure*. London: King's Fund.

Boardman, J., Henshaw, C. & Wilmott, S. (2004) Needs for mental health treatment among general practice attenders. *British Journal of Psychiatry,* **185**, 318-327.

Commission for Health Improvement (2003a) *What CHI has found in mental health trusts. Sector report*. London: Commission for Health Improvement.

Commission for Health Improvement (2003b) *Rating the NHS: NHS performance ratings 2002/2003*. Available from: http://www.chi.nhs.uk/eng/ratings/2003/index.shtml [Accessed 7 March 2005]

Department of Health (1989) *Working for Patients*. London: HMSO.

Department of Health (1999) *National Service Framework for Mental Health: Modern Standards and Service Models*. London: DH.

Department of Health (2004a) *Departmental Report 2004*. London: DH

Department of Health (2004b) *The National Service Framework for Mental Health – Five years on*. London: DH.

Department of Health (2004c) *NHS Reference Costs 2003 and National Tariff 2004*. London: DH.

Department of Health and Social Security (1986) *Public Expenditure on the Social Services: Memorandum submitted to the Social Services Select Committee 1985-86*. London: HMSO.

Forrest, E. (2004) The Right to Choose. *Health Service Journal*, 9 December 2004.

Glasby, J. & Lester, H. (2003a) *Hospital Services,* booklet 5 of *Cases for change: an overview of the evidence which is driving the agenda for change*. London: National Institute for Mental Health in England.

Glasby, J. & Lester, H. (2003b) *Forensic Services,* booklet 6 of *Cases for change: an overview of the evidence which is driving the agenda for change*. London: National Institute for Mental Health in England.

Glover, G. & Barnes, D. (2003) *Mental Health Service Provision for Working Age Adults in England 2002*. Durham: University of Durham/ National Institute for Mental Health in England.

Goldberg, D. & Huxley, P. (1992) *Common Mental Disorders*. London: Routledge.

Healthcare Commission (2004) *Rating the NHS: NHS performance ratings 2003/4*. London: Commission for Health Care Audit and Inspection. Available from: http://www.chi.nhs.uk/eng/ratings/index.shtml [Accessed 7 March 2005]

Levenson, R., Greatley, A. & Robinson, J. (2003) *London's State of Mind: King's Fund Mental Health Inquiry 2003*. London: King's Fund.

National Institute for Mental Health in England (2004) *Service Users and Carers: Latest Facts and Figures*. Available from: http://www.nimhe.org.uk/usersurvivor/facts.asp [Accessed 7 March 2005]

Office for National Statistics (2002) *Psychiatric Morbidity among Adults Living in Private Households, 2000.* London: The Stationery Office.

The Sainsbury Centre for Mental Health (2003a) *Money for Mental Health: A review of public spending on mental health care.* London: SCMH.

The Sainsbury Centre for Mental Health (2003b) *The Economic and Social Costs of Mental Illness.* Policy Paper 3. London: SCMH.

Social Exclusion Unit (2004) *Mental Health and Social Exclusion. Social Exclusion Unit Report.* London: ODPM.

Wanless, D. (2001) *Securing our Future Health: Taking a Long-term View. Interim Report.* London: HM Treasury.

Wanless, D. (2002) *Securing our Future Health: Taking a Long-term View. Final Report.* London: HM Treasury.

Chapter 6: From Little Acorns – The mental health service user movement

Crossley, N. (1999) Fish, field, habitus and madness: the first wave mental health users movement in Great Britain. *British Journal of Sociology,* **50** (4) 647-670.

Department of Health (1999) *National Service Framework for Mental Health: Modern Standards and Service Models.* London: DH.

Friedli, L. (2004a) Behind the scenes. *Mental Health Today,* July/August 2004, p14.

Friedli, L (2004b) Power to the people. *Mental Health Today.* October 2004, p14.

Good Practices in Mental Health/Camden Consortium (1988) *Treated Well? A code of practice for psychiatric hospitals.* London: GPMH.

House of Commons (1990) *The National Health Service and Community Care Act.* London: HMSO

Mental Health Foundation (2000) *Strategies for living: a report of user-led research into people's strategies for living with mental distress.* London: Mental Health Foundation.

Mental Health Foundation/The Sainsbury Centre for Mental Health (2002) *Being there in a crisis. A report of the learning from eight mental health crisis services.* London: Mental Health Foundation.

Openmind (2004) Bid for national take-up of ward round. *Openmind,* November/December 2004, p5.

Pembroke, L. (ed) (1994) *Self-harm: perspectives from personal experience.* London: Survivors Speak Out.

Read, J. & Baker, S. (1996). *Not Just Sticks and Stones: A survey of the discrimination experienced by people with mental health problems.* London: Mind.

Romme, M. & Escher, S. (1993) *Accepting Voices.* London: Mind.

Rose, D (2001) *Users' Voices: The perspectives of mental health service users on community and hospital care.* London: The Sainsbury Centre for Mental Health.

Social Exclusion Unit (2004) *Mental Health and Social Exclusion. Social Exclusion Unit Report.* London: ODPM.

Snow, R. (2002) *Stronger Than Ever: report of the 1st National Conference of Survivor Workers.* Stockport: Asylum.

Wallcraft, J., Read, J. & Sweeney, A. (2003) *On Our Own Terms: Users and survivors of mental health services working together for support and change.* London: The Sainsbury Centre for Mental Health.

Chapter 7: Primary Care and Mental Health

Balint, M. (1957) *The Doctor, His Patient, and The Illness.* London: Elsevier.

Cohen, A. (2004) *Practice-based Commissioning in the NHS.* London: The Sainsbury Centre for Mental Health. Available from: http://www.scmh.org.uk/8025695100388752/GenerateFrameset1?OpenAgent&doc=wpKHAL66LF25 [Accessed 7 March 2005]

Department of Health (1999) *National Service Framework for Mental Health: Modern Standards and Service Models.* London: DH.

Godber, G. (1975) *The Health Service: Past, Present and Future.* London: Athlone.

Moon, G. & North, N. (2000) *Policy and Place: General Medical Practice in the UK.* Basingstoke: Macmillan Press.

National Institute for Clinical Excellence (2004) *Anxiety: Management of anxiety (panic disorder, with or without agoraphobia, and generalised anxiety disorder) in adults in primary, secondary and community care. Clinical Guidance 22.* London: NICE.

Royal College of General Practitioners (1972) *The Future General Practitioner* London: RCGP

Social Exclusion Unit (2004) *Mental Health and Social Exclusion. Social Exclusion Unit Report.* London: ODPM.

Chapter 8: Mental Health Teams – Hitting the targets: missing the point?

Audit Commission (1986) *Making a Reality of Community Care.* London: HMSO.

Borrill, C. S., Carletta, J., Carter, A. J., Dawson, J. F., Garrod, S., Rees, A., Richards, A., Shapiro, D. & West, M. A. (2000) *The effectiveness of healthcare teams in the National Health Service.* Birmingham: Aston University.

Burns, T. (2004) *Community Mental Health Teams.* Oxford: OUP.

Clever, L. H. (1999) A call to renew. *British Medical Journal,* **319,** 1587-1588.

Chisholm, A. & Ford, R. (2004) *Transforming Mental Health Care: Assertive outreach and crisis resolution in practice.* London: SCMH.

Commission for Health Improvement (2003) *What CHI has found in mental health trusts. Sector report.* London: Commission for Health Improvement.

Corry, P., Drury, C.D. & Pinfold, V. (2004) *Lost and Found: Voices from the forgotten generation.* London: Rethink.

Dean, C., Phillips, E. M. Gadd, E. M., Joseph, M. & England, S. (1993) Comparison of community based service with hospital based service for people with acute, severe psychiatric illness. *British Medical Journal,* **307,** 473-476.

Department of Health (1999) *National Service Framework for Mental Health: Modern Standards and Service Models.* London: DH.

Department of Health (2000) *The NHS Plan: A plan for investment, a plan for reform.* London: DH.

Department of Health (2001) *The Mental Health Policy Implementation Guide.* London: DH.

Department of Health and Social Security (1988) *Report of the Committee of Inquiry into the Care and Aftercare of Miss Sharon Campbell.* London: HMSO.

Diamond, R. J. (1996) Coercion and tenacious treatment in the community: Applications to the real world. In: Dennis, D. L. & Monahan, J. (eds) *Coercion and aggressive community treatment. A new frontier in mental health law.* New York: Plenum Press.

Ford, R., Beadsmore, A., Ryan, P., Repper, J., Craig, T. & Muijen, M. (1995) Providing the safety net: case management for people with a serious mental illness. *Journal of Mental Health,* **1,** 91-97.

Health Service Journal (2004) *Psychiatrist examination.* 21st October 2004, p.29.

Healthcare Commission (2004) *Healthcare Commission Patient Survey.* London: Commission for Healthcare Audit and Inspection.

Hudson, B. (1996) Care management: Is it working? *Community Care Management and Planning,* **4** (3), 77-84.

Iles, V. & Sutherland, K. (2001) *Organisational Change.* London: NCCSDO.

Malone, B. (2004) Setting the scene. Presentation given at *Team Working Today* conference, Royal College of Nursing, 15th November 2004.

Marks, I. M., Connolly, J., Muijen, M., Audini, B., McNamee, G. & Lawrence, R. E. (1994) Home-based versus hospital-based care for people with serious mental illnesses. *British Journal of Psychiatry*, **165**, 179-194.

McAusland, T. (1985) *Planning and monitoring community mental health centres*. London: Kings Fund Centre.

McGuiness, M. (2004) Exploring the role of community mental health team managers. *Nursing Times*, **100** (32), 40-43.

Merson, S., Tyrer, P., Onyett, S., Lack, S., Birkett, P., Lynch, S. & Johnson, T. (1992) Early intervention in psychiatric emergencies: a controlled clinical trial. *The Lancet*, **339**, 1311-1314.

National Health Service Executive/Social Services Inspectorate (1999) *Effective care coordination in mental health services: Modernising the care programme approach.* London: DH.

National Institute for Mental Health in England (2004) *The Ten Essential Shared Capabilities – A framework for the whole of the mental health workforce.* London: DH.

National Institute for Mental Health in England (2005) *Guiding statement on recovery.* London: DH.

Onyett, S.R. (1992) *Case management in mental health.* Cheltenham: Stanley Thornes.

Onyett, S. R. (2003) *Teamworking in mental health.* Basingstoke: Palgrave

Onyett, S. R., Heppleston, T. & Bushnell, D. (1994) A national survey of community mental health teams. *Journal of Mental Health*, **3**, 175-194.

Onyett, S. R., Heppleston, T. & Muijen, M. (1995) *Making Community Mental Health Teams Work.* London. SCMH.

Onyett, S. R., Pillinger, T. & Muijen, M. (1997) Job satisfaction and burnout among members of community mental health teams. *Journal of Mental Health*, **6** (1) 55-66.

Patmore, C. & Weaver, T. (1991) *Community mental health teams: Lessons for planners and managers.* London: Good Practices in Mental Health.

Pendleton, D. & King, J. (2002) Values and leadership. *British Medical Journal*, **325**, 1352-1355.

Perkins, R. & Goddard, K. (2004) Reality out of the rhetoric: Increasing user involvement in a mental health trust. *Mental Health Review*, **9** (1).

Rankin, J. (2004) *Developments and Trends in Mental Health Policy.* London: Institute for Public Policy Research.

Richards, A. & Rees, A. (1998) Developing criteria to measure the effectiveness of community mental health teams. *Mental Health Care*, **21** (1) 14-17.

Rogers, A. & Pilgrim, D. (1993) Mental health service users' views of medical practitioners. *Journal of Interprofessional Care*, **7** (2) 167-176.

Rollnick, S. & Miller, W. R. (1995) What is motivational interviewing? *Behavioural and Cognitive Psychotherapy*, **23**, 325-334.

Rose, D., Ford, R., Lindley, P., Gawith, L. & The KCW Mental Health Monitoring Users' Group (1998) *In our experience: User-Focused Monitoring of Mental Health Services.* London: SCMH.

The Sainsbury Centre for Mental Health (2004a) *Briefing 27: Benefits and work for people with mental health problems.* London: SCMH.

The Sainsbury Centre for Mental Health (2004b) *Briefing 26: The Supporting People programme and mental health.* London: SCMH.

Sashidharan, S. P., Smyth, M. & Owen, A. (1999) PRiSM Psychosis Study: Thro' a glass darkly: A distorted appraisal of community care, *British Journal of Psychiatry*, **175**, 504-507.

Sayce, L., Craig, T. K. J. & Boardman, A. P. (1991) The development of community mental health centres in the UK. *Social Psychiatry and Psychiatric Epidemiology*, **26**, 14-20.

Wells, J. S. G. (1997) Priorities, 'street level bureaucracy' and the CMHT. *Health and Social Care in the Community*, **5** (5) 353-41

West, M. A. (1994) *Effective teamwork.* Leicester: BPS.

West, M. A. (2004) Building a team based future. Presentation given at *Team Working Today* conference, Royal College of Nursing, 15th November 2004.

West, M. A., Borrill, C. S., & Unsworth, K. L. (1998) Team effectiveness in organisations. In: Cooper, C. L. & Robertson, I. T. (eds). *International Review of Industrial and Organisational Psychology*. Chichester: John Wiley & Sons Ltd.

Chapter 9: The Social Context for Mental Health

Acheson, D. (1998) *Independent Inquiry into Inequalities in Health Report*. London: HMSO.

Advance Housing (2004) *Information leaflet 2004*. Available from: http://homeownershipdevelopment@advanceuk.org [Accessed 3 March 2005]

Bates, P. (ed) (2002) *Working for Inclusion: Making social inclusion a reality for people with mental health problems*. London: The Sainsbury Centre for Mental Health.

Becker, D.R., Bond G.R., McCarthy, D., Thompson, D., Xie, H., McHugo G.J. & Drake, R.E. (2001) Converting day treatment centers to supported employment programs in Rhode Island. *Psychiatric Services*, **52**, 351-357.

Berry, H.L. & Rickwood, D.J. (2000) Measuring social capital at the individual level: personal social capital, values and psychological distress. *International Journal of Mental Health Promotion*, **2** (3) 35-44.

Boardman, J. (2002) *Employment Opportunities and Psychiatric Disability*. Royal College of Psychiatrists Council Report (CR111). London: RCP.

Bond G.R., Drake, R.R., Mueser, K.T. & Becker, D.R (1997) An update on supported employment for people with severe mental illness. *Psychiatric Services*, **48** (3) 335-346.

Brugha, T.S., Wing, J.K., Brewin, C.R., MacCarthy, B. & Lasage, A. (1993) The relationship of social network deficits in social functioning in long term psychiatric disorders. *Social Psychiatry and Psychiatric Epidemiology*, **28**, 218-224.

Campbell, C. & McLean, C. (2002) Social capital, social exclusion and health: factors shaping African-Caribbean participation in local community networks. In: Health Development Agency. *Social capital for health: insights from qualitative research*. London: HDA

Campbell, C., Wood, R. & Kelly, M. (1999) *Social capital and health*. London: Health Education Authority.

Cohen, S (ed) (1997) *Measuring stress: a guide for health and social scientists*. Oxford: OUP.

Cooper, H., Arber, S., Fee, L. & Ginn, J. (1999) *The Influence of Social Support and Social Capital on Health*. London: HEA.

Department of Health (1999a) *General public attitudes to mental health/illness*. COI ref: RS4206. London: Central Office of Information.

Department of Health (1999b) *National Service Framework for Mental Health: Modern Standards and Service Models*. London: DH.

Department of Health (2000) *The NHS Plan: A plan for investment, a plan for reform*. London: DH.

Department of Health (2001) *Making it happen: a guide to developing mental health promotion*. London: DH.

Department of Health (2003) *Attitudes to mental illness 2003*. Available from: http://www.dh.gov.uk/PublicationsAndStatistics/Publications/PublicationsStatistics/PublicationsStatisticsArticle/fs/en?CONTENT_ID=4079111&chk=AVNPjX [Accessed 16 March 2005).

Department of Health (2004) *Choosing Health: Making healthy choices easier*. London: DH.

Dunn, S. (1999) *Creating accepting communities: report of the MIND inquiry into social exclusion and mental health problems* London: Mind

Gale, E. & Greatley, A. (2004) Turning public health on its head: The importance of mental health. In *ph.com: The Newsletter of the Faculty of Public Health,* June 2004.

Gale, E., Seymour, L., Crepaz-Keay, D., Gibbons, M., Farmer, P. & Pinfold, V. (2004) *Scoping Review on Mental Health and Anti-Stigma and Discrimination – current activities and what works.* Leeds: NIMHE.

Goffman, E. (1963) *Stigma: Notes on the management of spoiled identity.* London: Penguin Books.

Health Development Agency (2002) *Pre-retirement health checks and plans: literature review.* London: HDA.

Ion, R.M. & Beer, D. (2003) Valuing the past: The importance of an understanding of the history of psychiatry for healthcare professionals, service users and carers. *International Journal of Mental Health Nursing*, **12**, 237-242.

Jones, E., Farina, A., Hastorf, A., Markus, H., Miller, D. & Scott, R. (1984) *Social stigma: the psychology of marked relationships.* New York: Freeman.

Kawachi, I., Kennedy, B. & Lochner, K. (1997) Social Capital, Income Inequality and Mortality. *American Journal of Public Health*, **87**, 491-498.

Kawachi, I. & Kennedy, B.P. (1999) Income inequality and health: pathways and mechanisms. *Health Services Research*, **34**, 215.

Link, B. & Phelan, J. (2001) Conceptualising stigma. *Annual Review of Sociology,* **27**, 363-385.

Lister-Sharp, D., Chapman, S., Stewart-Brown, S. & Sowden, A. (1999) Health-promoting schools and health promotion in schools: two systematic reviews. *Health Technology Assessment*, **3** (22) 1-207.

Makkonen, T. (2003) *Main Causes, Forms and Consequences of Discrimination.* Available from: http://www.iom.fi/anti-discrimination/pdf/CH%20I%202003%20FINAL.pdf. [Accessed 2 March 2005]

Meltzer, H. (2003) *Further analysis of the Psychiatric Morbidity Survey 2000.* Data prepared for the Social Exclusion Unit. Unpublished.

Meltzer, H., Singleton, N., Lee, A., Bebbington, P., Brugha, T. & Jenkins, R. (2002) *The Social and Economic Circumstances of Adults with Mental Disorders.* London: The Stationery Office.

Mental Health Foundation (2000) *Strategies for living: report of user led research into people's strategies for living with mental distress.* London: Mental Health Foundation.

Mind (2004) *Not Alone? Isolation and Mental Distress.* London: Mind.

National Institute for Mental Health in England (2004) *From Here to Equality.* Leeds: NIMHE

Office for National Statistics *(2003) Quarterly Labour Force Survey, June-August 2003.* Available from: http://www.data-archive.ac.uk/findingData/snDescription.asp?sn=4751 [Accessed 2 March 2005]

Okun, M.A., Stock, W.A., Haring, M.J. & Witter, R.A. (1984) The social activity/subjective well-being relation: a quantitative synthesis. *Research on Ageing*, **6** (1) 45-65.

Oxman, T.E., Berkman, L.F., Karl, S., Freeman, D.H. & Barrett, J. (1992) Social support and depressive symptoms in the elderly. *American Journal of Epidemiology*, **135**, 356-368.

Read, J. & Baker, S. (1996) *Not Just Sticks and Stones: A survey of the discrimination experienced by people with mental health problems.* London: Mind.

Rethink (2003) *Just one per cent: What service users said about the current state of mental health provision in the UK.* London: Rethink Publications.

The Sainsbury Centre for Mental Health (2004) *Briefing 26: The Supporting People programme and mental health.* London: SCMH.

Sayce, L. (2000) *From Psychiatric Patient to Citizen: Overcoming discrimination and social exclusion.* Basingstoke: Macmillan.

Sayce, L. (2003) Beyond good intentions: making anti-discrimination strategies work. *Disability & Society*, **18** (5) 625-642.

Secker, J., Grove, B. & Seebohm P. (2001) Challenging barriers to employment, training and education for mental health service users: the service users perspective. *Journal of Mental Health*, **10** (4) 395-404.

Seebohm, P., Grove B. & Secker J. (2002) *Working Towards Recovery*. London: Institute for Applied Health and Social Policy.

Social Exclusion Unit (1998) *Rough Sleeping. Social Exclusion Unit Report*. London: Cabinet Office.

Social Exclusion Unit (2004) *Mental Health and Social Exclusion. Social Exclusion Unit Report*. London: ODPM.

Thomas, K., Secker J. & Grove, B. (2003) *Getting back before Christmas*. London: Institute for Applied Health and Social Policy.

Wanless, D. (2004) *Securing good mental health for the whole population: Final report*. London: DH.

Wilkinson, R. G. (1996) *Unhealthy Societies. The Afflictions of Inequality*. London: Routledge.

Wilkinson, R. (2000) Inequality and the social environment: a reply to Lynch *et al. Journal of Epidemiological Community Health*, **54**, 411-413.

Chapter 10: *Social Inequalities and Mental Health*

Acheson, D. (1998) *Independent Inquiry into Inequalities in Health: Report*. London: HMSO.

Appleyard, M. (2004) The Cinderella Trap. *The Independent,* 31 October.

Baker, S. (2000) *Environmentally Friendly? Patients' views of conditions on psychiatric wards*. London: Mind.

Ballou, M. & Brown, L. S. (eds) (2002) *Rethinking Mental Health and Disorder: Feminist Perspectives*. New York: Guilford.

Barron, J. (2004) *Struggle to Survive: Challenges for delivering services on mental health, substance misuse and domestic violence*. Bristol: Women's Aid Federation of England.

Beckett, C. & Macey, M. (2001) Race, gender and sexuality: the oppression of multiculturalism. *Women's Studies International Forum,* **24** (3/4), 309-2001.

Belle, D. & Doucet, J. (2003) Poverty, inequality, and discrimination as sources of depression among U.S. women. *Psychology of Women Quarterly,* **27** (2) 101-113.

Bertram, M. (2003) *Social inequalities, madness and the system: where are we?* Available from: http://psychminded.co.uk/ [Accessed 1 March 2005]

Bhui, K. (ed) (2002) *Racism and Mental Health*. London: Jessica Kingsley Publishers.

Burstow, B. (1992) *Radical Feminist Therapy: Working in the Context of Violence*. London: Sage.

Clancy, A., Hough, M., Aust, R. & Kershaw, C. (2001) *Crime, Policing and Justice: the Experience of Ethnic Minorities. Findings from the 2000 British Crime Survey*. London: Home Office.

Cogan, J. C. (1996) The prevention of anti-lesbian/gay hate crimes through social change and empowerment. In: Rothblum, E.D. & Bond, L.A. (eds) *Preventing Heterosexism and Homophobia*. London: Sage.

Cohen, L. J. (1994) Psychiatric hospitalization as an experience of trauma. *Archives of Psychiatric Nursing,* **8** (2) 78-81.

DeChant, B. (ed) (1996) *Women and group psychotherapy: Theory and practice*. New York: Guilford Press.

Department of Health (2002) *Women's Mental Health: Into the Mainstream – Strategic Development of Mental Health Care for Women*. London: DH.

Department of Health (2005) *Delivering Race Equality in Mental Health Care: An Action Plan for Reform Inside and Outside Services and The Government's Response to the Independent Inquiry into the Death of David Bennett*. London: DH.

Faulkner, A. & Layzell, S. (2000) *Strategies for Living: The Research Report*. London: Mental Health Foundation.

Fernando, S. (2003) *Cultural Diversity, Mental Health and Psychiatry: The Struggle Against Racism*. Hove, East Sussex: Brunner-Routledge.

Goater N., King, M., Cole, E., Leavey, G., Johnson-Sabine, E., Bhizad, R. & Hoar, A. (1999) Ethnicity and outcome of psychosis. *British Journal of Psychiatry*, **175** (1) 34 – 42

Harris, M. (2000) *Trauma Recovery and Empowerment: A Clinician's Guide for Working with Women in Groups*. London: Free Press.

Hollingshead, A. & Redlich, F. (1958) *Social class and mental illness*. New Haven, Connecticut: Yale University Press.

Humphreys, C. & Thiara, R. (2003) Mental health and domestic violence: 'I call it symptoms of abuse'. *British Journal of Social Work*, **33** (2) 209-226.

Kalikhat. (2004) Paying the price for not fitting in. *Asylum,* **14** (3) 26-27.

Keating, F. (2002). Black-led initiatives in mental health: An overview. *Research, Policy and Planning.,* **20** (2) 9-19

Keating, F., Robertson, D. & Kotecha, N. (2003) *Ethnic Diversity and Mental Health in London: Recent developments*. London: Kings Fund

King, M. & McKeown, E. (2003) *Mental health and social wellbeing of gay men, lesbians and bisexuals in England and Wales*. London: Mind Publications.

Martin, S. (2004) *A psychological understanding of mutual influence in men's abuse of female partners*. Canterbury: Tizard Centre, University of Kent.

Mental Health Media (2002) *What Women Want*. London: Mental Health Media.

Miller, J. & Bell, C. (1996) Mapping men's mental health. *Journal of Community and Applied Social Psychology*, **6** (5) 317-327.

National Institute For Mental Health In England (2003) *Inside Outside: Improving Mental Health Services for Black and Ethnic Minority Communities in England*. London: DH.

National Institute for Mental Health in England (2004) *The Ten Essential Shared Capabilities – A framework for the whole of the mental health workforce*. London: DH.

Nosek, M. A., Clubb, C. F., Hughes, R. B. & Howland, C. A. (2001) Vulnerabilities for abuse among women with disabilities. *Sexuality and Disability,* **19** (2) 177-189.

Penfold, P. S. & Walker, G. A. (1984) *Women and the Psychiatric Paradox*. Milton Keynes: Open University Press.

Pyke, N. (2004) Alan Bennett comes out fighting as he recounts the night he was beaten up. *The Independent on Sunday,* p. 12.

ReSisters (2002) *Women Speak Out*. Leeds: Leeds Women and Mental Health Action Group.

Rivera, M. (2002) The Chrysalis Program: A feminist treatment community for individuals diagnosed as personality disordered. In: Ballou, M. & Brown, L.S. (eds) *Rethinking Mental Health and Disorder: Feminist Perspectives*. New York: Guilford.

Rogers, A. & Pilgrim, D. (2003) *Mental Health and Inequality*. Basingstoke: Palgrave Macmillan.

The Sainsbury Centre for Mental Health (2002) *Breaking the Circles of Fear: A review of the relationship between mental health services and African and Caribbean communities*. London: SCMH.

Scott, S. & Williams, J. (2004) Closing the gap between evidence and practice: the role of training in transforming women's services. In: Jeffcote, N. & Watson, T. (eds) *Working Therapeutically with Women in Secure Mental Health Settings*. London: Jessica Kingsley.

Social Exclusion Unit (2004) *Mental Health and Social Exclusion. Social Exclusion Unit Report*. London: ODPM.

Tew, J. (ed) (2005) *Social Perspectives in Mental Health: Developing Social Models to Understand and Work with Mental Distress*. London: Jessica Kingsley.

Thornicroft, G., Davies, S. & Leese, M. (1999) Health service research and forensic psychiatry: A Black and White case. *International Review of Psychiatry*, **11** (2-3) 250-257.

Trivedi, P. (2002) Racism, social exclusion and mental health: A Black User's perspective. In: Bhui, K. (ed) *Racism and Mental Health*. London: Jessica Kingsley.

Wachtel, P. L. (2002) Psychoanalysis and the disenfranchised: From therapy to justice. *Psychoanalytic Psychology*, **19** (1) 199-215.

Waldrop, A. E. & Resick, P. A. (2004) Coping among adult female victims of domestic violence. *Journal of Family Violence*, **19** (5) 291-302.

Walters, V. & Charles, N. (1997) "I just cope from day to day": Unpredictability and anxiety in the lives of women. *Social Science and Medicine*, **45** (11) 1729-1739.

Weber, L. (1998) A conceptual framework for understanding race, class, gender, and sexuality. *Psychology of Women Quarterly*, **22**, 13-32.

White. A (2002) *Social Focus in Brief: Ethnicity*. London: Office for National Statistics.

Williams, J. (1999) Social inequalities, mental health and mental health services. In: Newnes, C. & Holmes, G. (eds) *Thinking About Psychiatry and The Future of the Mental Health System*. Ross-on-Wye: PCCS Books.

Williams, J. (2005) Women's Mental Health – Taking Inequality into Account. In: Tew, J. (ed) *Social Perspectives in Mental Health: Developing Social Models to Understand and Work with Mental Distress*. London: Jessica Kingsley.

Williams, J. & Keating, F. (2000) Abuse in mental health services: some theoretical considerations. *Journal of Adult Protection*, **2** (3) 32-39.

Williams, J., LeFrancois, B., & Copperman, J. (2001). *Mental Health Services that Work for Women: Survey Findings*. Canterbury: Tizard Centre, University of Kent.

Williams, J. & Scott, S. (2002) Service responses to women with mental health needs. *Mental Health Review*, **7** (1) 6-14.

Williams, J., Scott, S. & Bressington, C. (2004) Dangerous journeys: women's pathways through secure services. In: Jeffcote, N. & Watson, T. (eds) *Working Therapeutically with Women in Secure Settings*. London: Jessica Kingsley.

Websites

Equal Opportunities Commission [http://www.eoc.org.uk]

Department of Health (Publications and Statistics) [http://www.dh.gov.uk/PublicationsAndStatistics/fs/en]

Home Office (Research Development Statistics) [http://www.homeoffice.gov.uk/rds]

National Statistics [http://www.statistics.gov.uk]

Social Exclusion Unit [http://www.socialexclusionunit.gov.uk]

Fawcett Society [http://www.fawcettsociety.org.uk]

Commission for Racial Equality [http://www.cre.gov.uk]

Women's Aid [http://www.womensaid.org.uk]

Chapter 11: A View from Abroad – A new vision of stewardship

Bates, P. (ed) (2002) *Working for Inclusion: Making social inclusion a reality for people with severe mental health problems*. London: SCMH.

Department of Health (1998a) *Modernising Mental Health Services: Safe, Sound and Supportive*. London: DH.

Department of Health (1998b) *Modernising Social Services: Promoting independence, improving protection, raising standards*. London: DH.

Department of Health (1999) *National Service Framework for Mental Health: Modern Standards and Service Models*. London: DH.

Department of Health (2003) *Tackling Health Inequalities: A Programme for Action*. London: DH.

Department of Health and Human Services (1999) *Mental Health: A Report of the Surgeon General*. Rockville MD: DHHS.

Department of Health and Human Services (2001) *Culture, Race, and Ethnicity. Supplement to Mental Health: A Report of the Surgeon General.* Rockville MD: DHHS.

Department of Health and Human Services (2003) *Achieving the Promise: Transforming Mental Health Care in America. Final Report.* New Freedom Commission on Mental Health. Rockville MD: DHHS.

Drake, R.E. & Goldman, H.H. (2003) *Evidence-Based Practices in Mental Health Care.* Washington, D.C.: American Psychiatric Association

Glied, S. & Frank, R. (forthcoming) *Better, but not Well.* Baltimore, MD: The Johns Hopkins Press.

Hadley, T. & Goldman, H. (1995) The Effects of Recent Health and Social Services Policy Reforms on Britain's Mental Health System. *British Medical Journal,* **311,**1556-1558.

Hadley, T. & Goldman, H. (1998) A Partial Solution: A Local Mental Health Authority for the UK. *Journal of Mental Health Policy and Economics,* **1,** 73-76.

Kaiser Family Foundation (2004) *Employer Health Benefits 2004 Annual Survey.* Available from: www.kff.org/insurance/7148 [Accessed 22 February 2005]

Lehman, A.F., Goldman, H.H., Dixon, L.B. & Churchill, R. (2004) *Evidence-Based Mental Health Treatments and Services: Examples to Inform Policy.* New York: Milbank Memorial Fund. http://www.milbank.org/reports/2004lehman/2004lehman.html [Accessed 22 February 2005]

Mashaw, J.L. & Reno, V.P. (eds) (1996) *Balancing Security and Opportunity: The Challenge of Disability Income Policy. Report of the Disability Policy Panel.* Washington, D.C.: National Academy of Social Insurance.

The Sainsbury Centre for Mental Health (2002) *Breaking the Circles of Fear: A review of the relationship between mental health services and African and Caribbean communities.* London: SCMH.

The Sainsbury Centre for Mental Health (2003) *Money for Mental Health: A review of public spending on mental health.* London: SCMH.

Shepherd, G., Hadley, T., Muijen, M. & Goldman, H. (1996) The Impact of Mental Health Reforms on Clinical Practice in the UK: Back to the Future. *Psychiatric Services,* **47** (12) 1351-1355.

Shore, M. & Cohen, M. (1994) Introduction. *Millbank Quarterly,* **72** (1) 31-35.

Social Exclusion Unit (2004) *Mental Health and Social Exclusion. Social Exclusion Unit Report.* London: ODPM.

World Health Organization (2001) *The World Health Report. Mental Health: New Understanding, New Hope.* Geneva: World Health Organization.

Chapter 12: Afterword: From services to human rights

Department of Health (1999) *National Service Framework for Mental Health: Modern Standards and Service Models.* London: DH.

Department of Health (2004) *The National Service Framework for Mental Health – Five years on.* London: DH.

Roberts, G. & Wolfson, P. (2004) The Rediscovery of Recovery; open to all. *Advances in Psychiatric Treatment,* **10,** 37-49.

Wallcraft, J., Read, J. & Sweeney, A. (2003) *On Our Own Terms: Users and survivors of mental health services working together for support and change.* London: SCMH.

Woodbridge, K. & Fulford, K.W.M. (2004) *Whose Values? A workbook for values-based practice in mental health care.* London: SCMH.

World Health Organization (2005) *Mental Health Declaration for Europe.* Available from: http://www.euro.who.int/document/mnh/edoc06.pdf [Accessed 10 March 2005]